M000287175

OLYMPIC WEIGHTLIFTING FOR SPORTS

GREG EVERETT

CATALYST ATHLETICS

"Coach Everett's *Olympic Weightlifting for Sports* is an extraordinary product for any sport coach's library. As a proponent of the power clean and its variations for performance training, I found this book to be an outstanding reference for teaching methodology for the Olympic Movements. Coach Everett provides user-friendly terminology for the explanations of these movements. This book is a must-have for any coach who implements Olympic lifts in their program."
—*Joe Kenn, Head Strength and Conditioning Coach, Carolina Panthers*

"Coaches, make room on your bookshelf for Greg Everett's Olympic Weightlifting for Sports. Thorough, well written, well organized, and full of information & pictures to help make each point understandable. This will help make you a better coach, and in turn help improve your athletes' potential to succeed. I'm excited for Greg and excited to put the information to use!"
—*Jim Malone, Head Strength & Conditioning Coach, San Diego Padres*

"This is, by far, the most detailed and thorough book about Olympic weightlifting technique. Greg Everett has done an excellent job in presenting and organizing the material in this book. The photos are great. I strongly recommend that any strength coach or sports performance coach own this book if he/she is teaching deep squatting, snatch and clean pulls, and Olympic style lifts. It is well worth the money spent."
—*Ethan Reeve, Strength & Conditioning Coordinator, Wake Forest University*

"This book is a great addition to any strength & conditioning coach's library. It gives very basic and descriptive instruction that does not complicate what a strength & conditioning coach has to teach and coach on a daily basis regarding Olympic style lifts."
—*Kevin Yoxall, Head Strength & Conditioning Coach, Auburn University*

"Everett shows you how to utilize Olympic lifting as an incredibly safe and effective tool that improves the speed and quality of movement across all fields of athletics."
—*Eva Twardokens, two-time Olympian, World Championship bronze medalist, six-time national champion, 2011 USA Ski & Snowboard Hall of Fame inductee*

"*Olympic Weightlifting for Sports* is another outstanding book by Greg Everett that breaks down everything you need to know about the specifics of Olympic weightlifting. I really like the way Greg breaks down the progressions for each movement. I've always been a big believer in keeping things simple and specific for both coaches and athletes. This is a must-have for anyone trying to understand all aspects of Olympic lifting. All athletes need to understand why they are training a certain way. This book explicitly covers that for Olympic lifting."
—*Jeff Dillman, Director of Strength & Conditioning, University of Florida*

"Olympic Weightlifting for Sports is an excellent resource for coaches and athletes of all sporting venues. It provides detailed progressions and coaching cues to both effectively teach and learn the Olympic lifts with a mindset on sport utilization. A great addition to any individuals library looking to improve on the Olympic lifts in their program."
—*Jim McCarthy, Netherlands Olympic Speedskating Team*

"Greg Everett is my go-to resource when it comes to the Olympic lifts. Whether it's coaching, program design, or even addressing common limiting factors like flexibility, *Olympic Weightlifting for Sports* leaves no stone unturned. Whether you're a young coach learning the ropes or a grizzled veteran, this book is an amazing resource. Quite simply, if your goal is to teach athletes how to Olympic lift safely and effectively, this book needs to be in your library."
—*Mike Robertson, President of Robertson Training Systems and co-owner of Indianapolis Fitness and Sports Training*

"*Olympic Weightlifting for Sports* is a tremendous resource for strength coaches at all levels. Greg Everett covers all the necessary bases for developing an effective strength program with the incorporation of the Olympic lifts. Beginning and intermediate coaches will be able to learn the fundamentals, while advanced coaches will be able to examine some fresh thoughts and ideas on familiar training topics. All coaches and lifters involved in any form of strength training should have this book in their library."
—*Matt Foreman, Author of* Bones of Iron

Copyright 2012 Greg Everett

Published by Catalyst Athletics, Inc. All rights reserved. No part
of this book may be reproduced in any form without prior written
consent from the publisher.

ISBN-13 978-0-9800111-4-2
ISBN-10 0-9800111-4-0

APOD

Catalyst Athletics, Inc
www.catalystathletics.com

Catalyst Athletics, Inc and Greg Everett advise that the exercises
and techniques described in this book can be strenuous and may not
be appropriate for all individuals, and do not make any claim to the
safety of said exercises and techniques. The nutrition information
herein exists for example purposes only and in no way represents a
prescription for any individual. It is strongly recommended that the
reader consult a physician before engaging in any of the activities or
practices illustrated or described herein. Catalyst Athletics, Inc and
Greg Everett disclaim any and all liability for any injury sustained or
condition arising from the performance of any of the exercises or
practice of any of the nutrition ideas described in this book.

OLYMPIC WEIGHTLIFTING FOR SPORTS

GREG EVERETT

CATALYST ATHLETICS

CONTENTS

INTRODUCTION

The purpose of this book is simple: To provide athletes, coaches and trainers a straightforward and thorough resource to help them incorporate the Olympic lifts and their variants safely and effectively into training for sports other than competitive weightlifting. Most weightlifting books are intended for competitive weightlifters, including my own *Olympic Weightlifting: A Complete Guide for Athletes & Coaches*, leaving athletes and their coaches to figure out how to modify and apply the information to athletic goals different from maximal snatches and clean & jerks, and to contend with a level of detail that far surpasses what is necessary for their applications.

When training for a sport other than weightlifting, there is relatively little time available to dedicate to learning or teaching the lifts, and this is often as much a deterrent for their use by coaches and athletes as the complexity, perceived or real, of the lifts themselves. Additionally, many athletes arrive in programs that might otherwise incorporate the lifts without adequate preparation in terms of flexibility, trunk stability and basic motor patterns, leaving coaches and trainers wary of exposing them to the lifts.

My goal with this book is to provide all of the information a coach or athlete needs to teach or learn the Olympic lifts or certain variants both safely and effectively to allow them to capitalize on the benefits they provide with regard to the development of maximal athletic ability. The teaching progressions are intended to maximize effect and minimize time investment without sacrificing safety: to keep the entire approach as simple and straightforward as possible.

The inclusion of the Olympic lifts in some form will help athletes develop physical traits that improve the potential for performance in nearly any sport. With the help of this book, it's my hope that coaches and athletes will be confident enough to take advantage of the lifts and bring their training programs to the next level.

How to Use This Book

The book is split into topical sections that are organized to help the reader learn the necessary elements in a logical order. The first sections will provide an understanding of basic lift mechanics and considerations for ensuring athletes are properly prepared to perform the Olympic lifts. Next are teaching progressions for the Olympic lifts and the most useful variations in the recommended order of learning and implementation. Finally there is a brief discussion of program design and a section on improving flexibility specifically for the safe and effective performance of the Olympic lifts.

Throughout the teaching progressions for the lifts are summary boxes that provide simple and concise descriptions of the associated positions or drills. These can be used as quick reminders while learning or teaching, or they can be used instead of the more complete text initially to simplify as much as possible. However, it's recommended that the complete text be read and understood eventually, as it will add important details to the basics presented in the summary boxes.

THE FUNDAMENTALS

Definitions

The inconsistency of terminology with regard to the Olympic lifts within the athletic training community is probably attributable to the obscurity of the sport and the minimal interaction of weight-lifting coaches and weightlifters with coaches and athletes from other sports. Being able to communicate clearly is imperative for coaches to be able to share information and learn from each other. The following are quick explanations of the classic lifts and the primary variants or assistance exercises.

Snatch The snatch is the first of the two lifts contested in Olympic weightlifting. The athlete lifts the barbell from the floor to the overhead position in a single motion. The term snatch with no qualifiers implies a full squat in the bottom position.

Clean & Jerk The clean & jerk is the second of the two lifts contested in Olympic weightlifting. The athlete lifts the barbell first from the floor to the shoulders with the clean, and then from the shoulders to overhead with the jerk. The shorter movements and more advantageous positions allow athletes to lift more in the clean & jerk than in the snatch.

Clean In the clean, the athlete lifts the barbell from the floor to the shoulders. The term clean with no qualifiers implies a full squat in the bottom position.

Jerk There are three variations of the jerk: the split jerk, power jerk (or push jerk) and squat jerk. The split jerk is the most commonly used variation by competitive lifters. In the jerk, the athlete lifts the barbell from the shoulders in a standing position to overhead. The term jerk with no qualifiers implies the lifter's chosen jerk style: for weightlifters that will usually mean split jerk; for many athletes, it will mean a power or push jerk.

Split Jerk The most common jerk variation for weightlifters. The lifter receives the jerk in a split foot position.

Power (Push) Jerk The power jerk, or push jerk, is a jerk received with the feet in a squat position and the lifter at partial squat depth (The feet move in the power jerk and stay connected to the platform in the push jerk).

Squat Jerk The squat jerk is the least common jerk variation. The athlete receives the jerk in a full depth squat.

Power Snatch The power snatch is a snatch started from the floor but received overhead in a partial squat above parallel rather than a full squat.

Power Clean The power clean is a clean started from the floor but received on the shoulders in a partial squat above parallel rather than a full squat.

Hang Snatch The hang snatch is a snatch started with the bar in any position above the floor and received in a full squat position. The most common hang starting position is the bar just above the knees.

Hang Clean The hang clean is a clean started with the bar in any position above the floor and received in a full squat position. The most common hang starting position is the bar just above the knees.

Back Squat The back squat is often simply called the squat outside the weightlifting community where the need to distinguish it from the front squat is less common. This is a squat performed with the barbell racked on the shoulders behind the athlete's neck.

Front Squat The front squat is a squat performed with the barbell racked across the shoulders in front of the athlete's neck.

Overhead Squat The overhead squat is a squat performed with the bar held in locked arms overhead, most commonly with a snatch-width grip.

Snatch Pull The snatch pull is a training exercise that mimics the first phase of a snatch in which the bar is pulled with a snatch-width grip to complete hip and knee extension. The athlete does not make the attempt to relocate the body underneath the bar, but there is an effort to accelerate the bar maximally. A snatch high-pull involves a continued pull with the arms after the legs and hips have extended.

Clean Pull The clean pull is a training exercise that mimics the first phase of a clean in which the bar is pulled with a clean-width grip to complete hip and knee extension. The athlete does not make the attempt to relocate the body underneath the bar, but there is an effort to accelerate the bar maximally. A clean high-pull involves a continued pull with the arms after the legs and hips have extended.

Press The press is a strength exercise in which the athlete lifts the barbell from the shoulders to overhead exclusively with the upper body.

Push Press The push press is a press that begins with a dip and drive of the legs to accelerate the barbell upward before the upper body engages to finish the push of the barbell into the overhead position.

How & Why the Olympic Lifts Work

The snatch, clean and jerk can all be split into two basic phases. First is the effort of the athlete to accelerate the barbell upward maximally by explosively driving against the floor with the legs and extending the hips (the jerk is a drive with the legs only). Second is the effort of the athlete to aggressively pull (or push in the jerk) the body down against the barbell to receive it either overhead in the snatch and jerk or on the shoulders in the clean. The first phase is easily understood and practiced; the second is more commonly misunderstood and incorrectly performed. With heavy weights, the athlete cannot simply drop under the bar; there must be an active and aggressive effort to change the body's direction at the end of the first phase and relocate underneath the weight.

There are three basic elements to the Olympic lifts' benefit to athletic ability. The first is the most obvious: the improvement of knee and hip extension power (power is the combination of strength and speed; we can also call this explosiveness) and rate of force development. This element is trained during the first phase (primarily during the final explosive effort starting when the bar reaches the level of approximately mid-thigh).

The second element is the improvement of an athlete's ability to safely and effectively absorb force or decelerate. This is trained to some degree with basic strength work such as squatting, but the nature of receiving the barbell in the Olympic lifts is far more ballistic and more similar to the demands on ground-based athletes with regard to stopping, changing direction or absorbing the force of colliding opponents.

The third element is the collective improvement of kinesthetic awareness, fundamental athletic motor skills centered around the hips and legs, and the precise and consistent control of body positions and movements.

No other exercises provide training for these things to the same degree, particularly so efficiently.

The Role of the Olympic Lifts in Athletic Training

All athletes must possess a set of physical skills and characteristics specific to their sport and occasionally even more specifically to their position within that sport. These skill sets can vary broadly among sports and athletes, but few athletes will not benefit from improving strength, particularly in the lower body, speed, explosiveness and the ability to safely and productively absorb force.

Some sports demand a great amount of time to be dedicated to sport-specific skill, leaving comparatively little time for strength and conditioning; other sports, generally because of a more limited number of skills or skill types, allow for and even demand more time to be dedicated to strength and conditioning. Obviously the more power and strength oriented a sport, the larger the role strength and power training will play in the training of the athlete. Arguably the best example of this would be the thrower, who focuses on as little as a single discipline (e.g. discuss, shot, hammer), and whose success depends heavily on strength and power. Strongman competitors are clearly in need of a great deal of strength, but also must be possessed of considerable stamina and a fair number of skills. Football players also have considerable need for strength, speed and power, but also need to develop to a high level conditioning and a fairly wide array of skills. The endurance athlete has the least need for strength and power development, but will unquestionably still benefit from training these qualities to the appropriate extent.

When designing strength and conditioning programs for any athlete, it's necessary to understand the actual needs of the athlete in terms of the demands of the sport and the present state of athletic development of the individual. What is appropriate and effective for one athlete may be far from it for another.

In some cases, the Olympic lifts will not be appropriate because an athlete does not have adequately developed foundational abilities in terms of strength, flexibility and basic athletic movement patterns; in other cases it may impossible to incorporate the lifts because of severe time or equipment limitations and the need to prioritize both training time and training effect. In instances of power athletes training full time, the Olympic lifts may play a significant role and appear both frequently and in relatively high volume in the training program.

Ultimately the role of the Olympic lifts will be determined based on the needs and circumstances of each athlete.

Technical Differences of the Lifts for Athletic Training

There are certain subtle details of the technical performance of the Olympic lifts that may vary in necessity or appropriateness when comparing athletes to competitive weightlifters. The exclusive goal of the weightlifter is to snatch and clean & jerk as much weight as possible, and technique will be shaped to meet that end. However, the athlete using the lifts for another sport is interested in developing certain physical traits that will carry over into athletic performance outside the gym, not directly in the amount of weight lifted.

The primary distinction that should be made is that for the athlete, minimizing the risk of injury in the weightroom is paramount. Moreover, training in the weightroom should contribute to the athlete's ability to withstand injury on the field. With this in mind, performing the lifts with the safest possible positions takes priority over possible departure from this merely for the sake of lifting more weight. A simple example is the squat: The competitive weightlifter must squat to absolute maximal depth in order to get under as much weight as possible. Occasionally this involves less than ideal mechanics at the knee or hip that for the weightlifter are worth the risk, but for other athletes are not. This may somewhat limit what an athlete is capable of lifting, but again, the weight itself is not the goal.

Among competitive weightlifters of any level, there are variations in technical style. Generally these are subtle enough to not be noticeable to individuals not steeped in the culture of weightlifting. The pertinent example is the dominance of hip extension over knee extension of some lifters to the extent that the development of knee extension power is limited. While this can be an effective strategy for certain lifters for whom it allows a faster transition under the bar, it's not appropriate for athletes interested in optimally developing lower body explosiveness that will transfer maximally to performance in their chosen sports. What is presented technically in this book does not necessary represent what would be taught to a competitive lifter: it is specifically intended to provide the most possible benefit to athletes of different sports.

Safety of the Olympic Lifts

Commonly coaches and parents of young athletes are under the impression that lifting weights is dangerous, and Olympic weightlifting appears to be particularly injurious based on casual observation or rumor.

In fact, Olympic weightlifting is remarkably safe, and the injury rate among competitive weightlifters is extremely low—far lower than the more conventional sports parents are more than happy to let their kids participate in. All sport has the potential for injury, particularly at high levels of competition. However, the overwhelming majority of weightlifting injuries are incurred by individuals with little or no instruction in the lifts who are training improperly in terms of technique, loading and program design. It should be no surprise that athletes with inadequate mobility can hurt themselves trying to perform lifts that demand considerable mobility; nor should it be a surprise that athletes injure themselves pushing lifts beyond their technical abilities, whether in competition with each other or themselves.

According to a chart from the International Weightlifting Federation[1], the number of injuries per 100 participant hours for weightlifting in the UK was 0.0017[2]. Compare this to American Football, which had 0.100; US Track & Field, which had 0.570; or US Basketball, which had 0.030.

In any case, the Olympic lifts are no riskier than any other strength & conditioning activity if instructed, coached, performed and programmed properly. It's the responsibility of the coach and athlete to ensure safety in the weight room regardless of the training modality.

---

1 International Weightlifting Federation: www.iwf.net
2 There was no figure for weightlifting in the US available. Presumably participation is too low.

EVALUATION

A proper evaluation of each athlete will help guide the design of the training program appropriately. The demands of the athlete's sport and the circumstances in which the athlete will be training will influence the details of the program. The goal of all program design is to maximize effectiveness within the allowable time and with the available resources. Time and resources can vary widely among coaches and athletes, and as a consequence, programs may look dramatically different, yet all of these programs may be considered optimal.

Sport Evaluation

The most basic step in designing a training program is determining the demands of the sport. Basic athletic characteristics can be prioritized to ensure the appropriate amount of time and effort is given to each element. These characteristics are:

- Strength
- Speed
- Power (explosiveness)
- Cardiorespiratory Endurance
- Stamina (local muscular endurance)
- Flexibility/Mobility

This list does not take into consideration sport-specific skills; it includes only fundamental abilities that can be trained primarily in the gym.

Athlete Evaluation

General Athletic Assessment Each athlete should be assessed for basic athletic qualities such as strength, speed, stamina, endurance and power. This list will vary somewhat depending on the demands of the sport. Each aspect should be prioritized, at least informally, based on the combination of the sport's demand and the athlete's present state of development. For example, for a given athlete, strength may not be the first priority with regard to the sport itself, but it may be the area in which the athlete is least developed and therefore it should be prioritized within the training plan.

Basic Strength Movement Proficiency Any athlete wishing to incorporate the Olympic lifts or their variants into a training program should have an established foundation of basic strength movements. Without such a foundation, athletes will typically not be able to use the Olympic lifts effectively both because it will be a much longer and more involved process to learn them, but also simply because they will be unable to use loading adequate to provide a significant training stimulus.

Athletes should be familiar with the squat, deadlift and press at minimum. Those who are not but who are interested in learning the Olympic lifts would be well served spending at least a short amount of time learning these basic strength exercises first. Assessing an athlete's proficiency on these exercises should be done primarily based on mechanics and secondarily on loading; an athlete's strength in a given exercise is not necessarily reflective of movement quality.

Flexibility & Mobility The Olympic lifts require a certain degree of mobility in the ankles, hips, upper back, shoulders and wrists. Easily the most common limiter on the performance of the lifts is inadequate flexibility. Athletes with flexibility limitations may need to employ variations of the lifts that demand less flexibility, such as power cleans or power snatches, or limitations may be correctable quickly enough that the athlete can, after a brief preparation period, use the full lifts if so desired. Adequate flexibility will play a significant role in safety both with regard to the Olympic lifts and basic strength lifts.

Flexibility can be measured for the Olympic lifts best with certain movements and positions rather than direct flexibility testing. The following movements and positions should be tested:

- Olympic Back Squat
- Front Squat
- Overhead Squat
- Jerk Rack Position
- Jerk Overhead Position

An athlete's ability or inability to achieve the necessary positions in the previous tests will tell the coach which exercises are immediately accessible and which will require improvements in flexibility before being possible or safe. See the Flexibility chapter of the book for more information on evaluating and correcting flexibility.

Injury History & Limitations Before starting any training program, an athlete's injury history should be considered and any limitations arising from past injuries taken into account. This may encourage the coach to use somewhat different exercises to avoid re-injury or aggravation of an existing injury, or to modify movements due to range of motion restrictions.

Circumstance Evaluation

Time How much time will the athlete be able to dedicate to training in total, to strength & conditioning generally, and to the Olympic lifts specifically? For high school athletes in particular, training time is typically limited due to facility use and staff issues. In these cases, coaches often need to be creative and focus on efficiency when designing the training program. For non-scholastic athletes, training time may be limited instead by obligations such as work and family, or due to financial restrictions.

Facility & Equipment How much space and what equipment is available to the athlete and coach? If working with large groups of athletes, are there an adequate number of barbells, racks, platforms and weights? If working as an individual athlete, is weightlifting equipment available as well as space in a facility that allows such use of the equipment?

Staff For professional or semi-professional coaches working with large numbers of athletes, are there an adequate number of qualified staff members to assist in teaching and coaching in the weight room to ensure that athletes are performing the lifts safely and effectively?

TEACHING PROGRESSIONS

The goal for the following teaching progressions is to teach athletes to perform the lifts as quickly and easily as possible without compromising safety or effectiveness. Some athletes will naturally learn the movements more quickly than others. Certain athletes may require additional drills to help perform the movements more accurately; others will simply need a greater volume of repetition.

It's important to remember that we are not producing competitive weightlifters. Athletes do not need to perform the Olympic lifts with technical perfection. However, the more proficient they are, the more they will benefit from training the lifts, and the safer that training will be.

After the initial learning stage, athletes should be encouraged to remain focused on technical execution every time they train the lifts to continually improve over time rather than allowing suboptimal technique to become habit. If time allows, a few minutes of technique practice can be done as part of the warm-up before Olympic lift training to allow athletes the chance to fine-tune their movements over time.

Despite being taught a standard technical execution of the lifts, every athlete will look somewhat different performing them. This variation will arise from factors such as individual body proportions, innate speed and timing capabilities and the extent of technique development at any given time. It's important for the coach to be able to distinguish between such acceptable variation and divergence from safe and effective technique. In no instance should an athlete be allowed to continue performing a lift in an unsafe manner.

GREG EVERETT

Teaching Order

The following progression is the suggested order of teaching the lifts whether all or only some are taught. The hang-power variations of the clean and snatch are taught before the power variations from the floor, both because this is the ideal way to teach them, and also because it's likely that many athletes will exclusively lift from the hang. Power variations are taught before squat variations because the power lifts will deliver the most benefit generally to athletes and are also far less demanding on flexibility.

The power clean is first because it's the simplest Olympic lift variation for leg and hip explosiveness, yet still very effective. The push press and jerk follows to provide exercises involving some upper body pushing power to complement the lower body power development of the power clean; the push press and jerk are also typically easier to learn for athletes than the snatch. The power snatch follows the push press and jerk because of its greater difficulty, and because of its lesser comparative necessity and utility if the athlete is already performing power cleans. The squat variations from the floor are last because they are the most demanding of flexibility, and will likely never be used by most athletes, both because the time needed to develop them may be more than what is available, and because the benefits they offer over the power variations are not proportionate to the time needed to develop the technique and flexibility.

This order of learning the lifts will also allow athletes to begin implementing some form of Olympic lifting as quickly as possible if developing adequate flexibility to perform the full classic lifts is necessary.

1. Hang Power Clean
2. Power Clean
3. Push Press
4. Power Jerk
5. Split Jerk
6. Hang Power Snatch
7. Power Snatch
8. Clean
9. Snatch

Loading

The following drills are intended to be performed with an empty barbell. Some athletes may need to use lighter technique barbells for certain drills.

Sets and Repetitions

The following learning progressions are comprised of brief drills intended to teach specific portions of the whole movements while being simple and easy both for coaches to instruct and athletes to learn. Numbers have not been prescribed—this is a flexible teaching system that can be adjusted according to the needs of the athlete or circumstances in a group or team setting.

Generally speaking, more repetitions are better than fewer, assuming the quality of those repetitions remains as high as possible. However, sets should be limited to 5 reps, even when working with empty barbells. Skill work is deceptively difficult even at very light weights and can be mentally exhausting. Each set needs to be performed as well as possible, and athletes can't be expected to perform optimally if fatigued.

Coaches and athletes can determine the appropriate or necessary volume of repetitions for each drill. This determination should be based simply on how well the athlete performs the drill. In most cases, athletes should be able to move through the series of drills and begin performing the exercise itself in a single training session. That being said, there is nothing wrong with extending the drill period if it appears to be necessary or beneficial, or to return to some or all of the drills as needed. The same drills used for learning and teaching the lifts initially will also be effective technique drills for athletes already performing the lifts but needing improvement in execution.

A simple example, using the hang power clean to illustrate, would be to perform 3-5 sets of 5 repetitions of each drill. If an athlete struggles with any particular drill, more time should be spent on it; similarly, if at athlete performs a drill perfectly on the first set, there is no need to spend more time on it.

Breathing and Trunk Pressurization

With all structural loading, athletes need to properly pressurize the trunk to establish spinal stability. This is critical for both performance and safety. To properly stabilize the trunk, the athlete needs to expand the abdomen and draw in a full breath. With the breath locked in, the athlete will tighten the abdominal and back musculature forcefully. The abs should not be drawn in or hollowed, as this simply narrows the base of support and decreases stability.

This breath should be taken prior to the initiation of a lift and held for the duration of a rep, excepting a controlled release of a small amount of air during the most difficult segment of a lift. For example, during the recovery of a heavy squat, air can be released as the lifter fights through the sticking point. The key is that only a small quantity should be released while maintaining a tight trunk, generally necessitating some noise with the expulsion.

Any time an athlete feels dizzy or lightheaded during a lift, the lift should be stopped immediately and safely and the athlete should sit down to recover.

The Hook Grip

Weightlifters, when snatching and cleaning, use the hook grip to increase grip security during the explosive acceleration of the lifts. Some athletes will not need to use the hook grip, but all are encouraged to learn it and use it to prevent grip strength from becoming a limiter of the Olympic lifts.

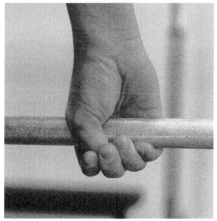

The athlete will press the skin between the thumb and index finger into the bar, then wrap the thumb around the bar as much as possible. The fingers will then be closed around the bar. The

The hook grip

index and middle fingers will be over the thumb: they should pull the thumb farther around the bar as the hand as a whole grips it.

The hook grip will be uncomfortable if not painful initially. Athletes will need to spend some time using it for the hand to become adequately mobile. The learning stages are ideal for this because the weight on the bar will be limited, which will minimize discomfort. The thumb can be taped with elastic athletic tape if necessary.

THE SQUAT

While not an Olympic lift itself, the squat is foundational to the lifts and is a staple strength training exercise. For athletes who will be performing only the power variations of the Olympic lifts, the full squat will not be necessary; however, the squat is discussed here to ensure athletes and coaches are completely prepared if they choose to use the full lifts. Additionally, even power receiving positions are squats in essence—they are simply partial depth squats. The foot position for the squat as described below is the same position in which athletes should receive all lifts, whether power or squat depth (with the exception of the split jerk).

The placement of the feet will dictate how the athlete is able to move in the squat, and this will determine whether or not the squat can be safe. The purpose of the correct stance is to ensure that the knees are hinging properly rather than experiencing rotation, and that the hips are able to move unimpeded through the necessary range of motion to achieve the full depth with a sound spine position.

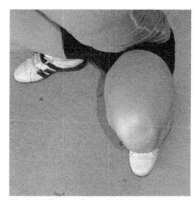

The width of the feet and how much the toes are turned out will be determined by each individual's proportions and mobility. What is necessary is that at any point during the squat, each thigh is parallel to its corresponding foot; in other words, the knee is hinging properly.

The thigh and foot should be approximately parallel with each other when viewed from directly above with the knee over the foot (not inside or outside of the foot).

Squat Position

- Feet hip to shoulder width
- Toes turned out 10-30 degrees
- Thigh parallel with foot in bottom position
- Feet flat, weight toward heels
- Back arched and trunk tight

The toes should be turned out between about 10-30 degrees to allow the hips to open properly as the athlete squats down. If the toes are directed forward, the thighs must also be directed forward to maintain proper knee mechanics; this position will not allow most athletes to maintain the proper arch in their backs, and will also force them to lean farther forward as they squat.

A simple way to find the proper squat stance is to simply place the feet just outside hip width and sit into a relaxed squat position. From this bottom position, the width and angle of the feet should be adjusted until the athlete finds a comfortable angle for the hips that also allows the thigh to be parallel with the foot.

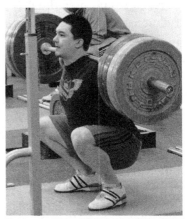

Minimum depth for the squat is just below parallel—that is, the crease of the hips is below the top of the knee. When performing the Olympic lifts, ideal depth is achieved when the knee joint is closed as much as possible with the maintenance of complete back extension. Based on how lifters are built, this absolute depth will appear different.

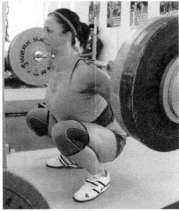

Athletes with shorter upper legs (top) will not be able to sit as low as athletes with longer upper legs and good flexibility (bottom).

For safe squatting, the minimum requirement is that the athlete maintain a neutral curvature of the spine. This requires a reasonable degree of hip and ankle mobility that may not be present in many athletes initially. It is strongly recommended that squats not be loaded with significant weight if an athlete is unable to maintain this arch of the back throughout the full range of motion.

The athlete's weight should be balanced across the foot with a slight preference for the heel. The squat should be performed with simultaneous movement of the knees and hips to allow the maintenance of a relatively upright trunk throughout the movement.

The Back Squat

The back squat is the most basic squat variation. The barbell is placed behind the neck between the top of the traps and the top of the shoulders. The shoulder blades should be squeezed back tightly and the bar placed on the bulk of the traps, not in contact with the bones of the neck. A narrower grip on the bar will help this position as well as help keep the upper back extended properly. The elbows should be oriented down—lifting them up and back will encourage the chest to drop forward and the upper back to round.

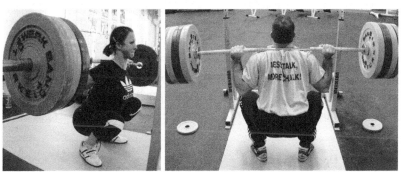

Correct placement of the barbell for the back squat

HANG POWER CLEAN

Our first lift is the hang power clean. This is the simplest and most accessible Olympic lift variation, and if an athlete never moves beyond it, he or she will still have a very effective training tool for lower body explosiveness and force absorption. This is also an excellent foundation to learning the rest of the lifts.

STEP 1 Rack Position

Likely the most important element of ensuring safety for athletes when performing the power clean or clean is the rack position, the position in which the athlete will receive the barbell on the shoulders at the completion of the lift. If done properly, this will be a comfortable, secure position; if done improperly, it will place excessive strain on the wrists and elbows in particular.

The first and most important thing to understand about the rack position is that the barbell is supported on the shoulders, not in the hands and arms. The shoulders are pushed forward and slightly up (scapular protraction and some elevation) to create space be-

---

1 Rack Position
- Grip wider than the shoulders
- Shoulders pushed forward and slightly up
- Bar between the peak of the deltoids and the throat
- Hands open and only the fingers under the bar
- Elbows high

---

tween the peak of the deltoid and the throat for the bar to rest in. The upper back should remain as extended as possible rather than rounded forward with the protraction of the shoulder blades. The hands are open and relaxed with only the ends of the fingers under the bar and the heel of the palm above the bar. Most athletes will rack the clean with only the first three fingers under the bar. It may require stretching to achieve this position comfortably.

A starting point for grip width is a half a fist-width to a full fist-width outside the shoulders. This somewhat wider grip will allow better positioning on the shoulders for most athletes, as well as bring the bar higher up on the thighs during the explosion phase of the lift and allow a quicker and mechanically sounder turnover. Ultimately each athlete will need to experiment to find the grip width that suits him or her best. The fingers should never be between the bar and shoulders and there should be no pain aside from initial discomfort due to inflexibility.

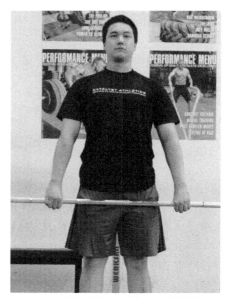

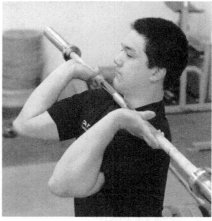

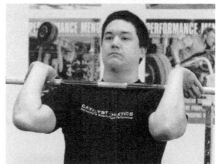

Top: Clean grip width;
Bottom: clean rack postion

STEP 2 Hang Position

The hang power clean will begin in a position with the bar just above the knees. The feet should be in the pulling position—approximately hip width or slightly wider with the toes turned out somewhat. With the proper clean grip on the bar, the athlete will set the back tightly in an arch, hinge at the hips, unlocking the knees and sliding the bar down the thigh until it stops just above the kneecaps.

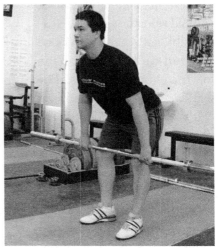

Clean hang position

In this position, the shins and arms should be vertical, the back arched tightly with the head and eyes straight forward, the points of the elbows turned to the sides (upper arm internally rotated), and the weight somewhat behind mid-foot (more pressure on the heels than on the balls of the feet, but still full foot contact with the floor). As part of the effort to maintain a proper back arch, the lats should be engaged, and this will help push the barbell back toward the body as the athlete extends.

---

2 Hang Position

- Feet hip width and toes turned out slightly
- Shins and arms approximately vertical
- Bar just above knee
- Weight toward heels
- Back arched and head forward
- Elbows pointed to the sides

GREG EVERETT

STEP 3 Jump & Bump

The "jump & bump" is the explosion phase of the power clean: the violent extension of the knees and hips to accelerate the barbell upward. At this point, underscoring that this acceleration is accomplished exclusively by the lower body is important. Understanding this at the outset will prevent some of the most common errors in the performance of the clean and snatch (and even jerk) and will help ensure that the athlete is reaping maximum benefit from the lift.

Before adding speed to this drill, the athlete will first do a slow movement to feel the proper positions. Starting in the hang position, the athlete will start by pushing against the floor with the legs, keeping the barbell as close to the thighs as possible without contacting them. When the bar reaches approximately mid-thigh, the athlete will extend the hips as the knees continue extending. The bar should come into contact with the upper thighs as the athlete completes the combined hip and knee extension through the active push back of the bar into the body with the lats. In this final extended position, the athlete's weight should be more on the heels than the balls of the feet, the bar touching the upper thighs at arms' length, the points of the elbows still turned to the sides, the knees straight and the hips very slightly hyperextended, placing the shoulders slightly behind the hips.

It's important that this small degree of hyperextension is actually occurring at the hip, not in the lumbar spine. To ensure this, the glutes should be activated to extend the hip and the abs kept tight to help maintain proper spine position.

When this basic movement is done properly, the balance maintained correctly over the foot, the bar contacting at the upper thigh, and the finish position achieved with proper glute activation,

---

3 Jump & Bump
- Start in the hang position
- Push against the floor with the legs
- Jump and extend the hips completely
- Push the bar against the upper thighs

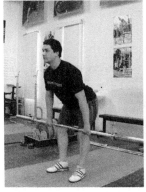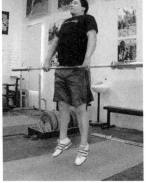

Jump & Bump

the athlete will move on to the full-speed drill.

From the hang starting position, the athlete will initiate the movement with the same push of the legs against the floor, then jump as the bar reaches mid-thigh level, extending the hips completely while pushing the bar back against the upper thighs with the lats. The goal at this point is not to do a maximal vertical jump, but to feel the concerted explosion of knees and hips with proper contact of the bar against the body.

During this movement, the athlete's arms should remain as relaxed as possible, being extended only by the weight of the barbell pulling on them. As the jump is completed, the bar should be kept in tight against the body, not allowed to bounce off the legs and swing forward. The athlete's feet should be landing on the floor in the same place they started; moving forward or backward indicates that the athlete's balance is starting or shifting too far in the direction of movement.

STEP 4 Pull

The pull drill is the first part of the second phase of the lift: the athlete's active pull of the body down under the barbell to receive it. This is an often neglected element of the Olympic lifts by athletes and coaches, but it's necessary both to help ensure a complete, and therefore safe, turnover, as well as allow the athlete to lift as much weight as he or she is truly capable of. This is literally an acceleration of the athlete's body down under the bar.

Standing tall with the feet in the same position used in the

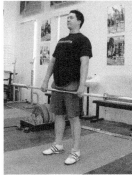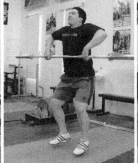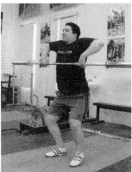

Pull

hang start, the athlete will make sure the points of the elbows are turned to the sides and the weight is more on the heels than the balls of the feet. Simultaneously, the athlete will pull down against the bar with the arms and jump the feet out into the squat position, squatting partially down with the effort to pull against the bar. The elbows should move up and out to the sides, keeping the barbell and body in immediate proximity to each other, with the chest up rather than leaning down to the bar. Typically athletes will perform this drill better if they think of moving the feet first before initiating the pull with the arms. If the athlete tries to perform them together, the arms will usually lead significantly.

The movement of the feet should be quick and aggressive, with minimal elevation—they should leave the floor only enough to be moved out to the squat stance and reconnected flat with aggression. This separation ensures that there is no pressure against the floor initially when the athlete is accelerating downward, and allows the feet to contact the floor completely flat, which will help ensure they are positioned under the athlete's center of mass. It may help the athlete to think of punching the heels back down into the floor.

---

4 Pull

- Start standing tall in the pulling position
- Pull down against the bar with the arms
- Jump the feet to the squat position and sit into a partial squat
- Elbows move up and to the sides

STEP 5 Rack

The rack delivery drill allows the athlete to practice the proper mechanics of a smooth and accurate delivery of the bar onto the shoulders, which is critical to successful and safe cleans. The two most important points here are that the bar should come into contact with the shoulders smoothly without crashing down onto them, and that the bar must be immediately secured on the shoulders in the proper high-elbow and open-hand rack position.

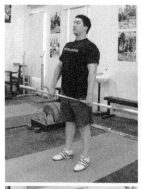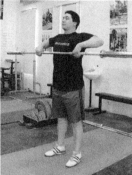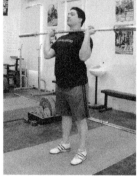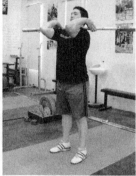

Rack

Standing tall, the athlete will turn the points of the elbows to the sides and ensure the weight is balanced on the foot toward the heel. The elbows should be pulled up and to the sides as high as possible, with the bar in immediate proximity to the body. As the elbows reach this maximum height, the bar should be pulled back

---

5 Rack

- Pull the elbows up and to the sides
- Spin the elbows around the bar
- Bring the shoulders up and forward to support the bar
- Relax the hands as the bar comes to rest on the shoulders and the elbows finish rising

---

GREG EVERETT

as the elbows are spun around the bar, guiding the bar to the shoulders smoothly. The grip on the bar should be maintained until the elbows have moved around under the bar and begin rising; at this point, the bar should be resting on the shoulders and the hands will be able to open as needed without the bar moving out of place.

This drill can be performed relatively slowly initially if needed to ensure proper elbow movement and a smooth connection of the bar to the shoulders. Eventually the whip of the elbows around the bar needs to be extremely quick.

STEP 6 Hang Power Clean

The final step in the progression is the hang power clean. This is simply the assembly of the previous steps into a single fluid movement: Jump & bump, pull & rack. Initially the movement should be practiced with an empty barbell as the previous drills were. This

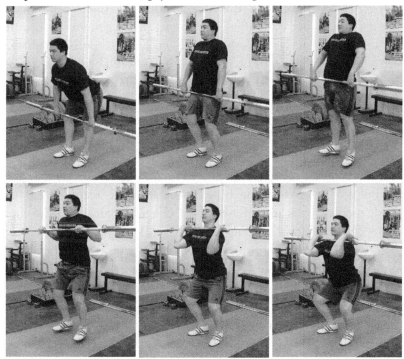

Hang power clean

6 Hang Power Clean

- Start in the hang position
- Push against the floor with the legs
- Extend the hips explosively with continued leg drive
- Push the bar back into the upper thighs with the lats
- Jump the feet out to the squat position
- Pull down against the bar with the elbows high and to the sides
- Spin the elbows around the bar and relax the grip

will require conscious control of the power put into the movement. At this point, the goal is to develop control over the movement of the body and barbell, and part of this is knowing how much force to apply.

From the hang position, the athlete will start with a push of the legs against the floor. As the bar reaches mid-thigh, he or she will explode with the hips while continuing to punch against the floor with the legs, using the lats to push the bar back into the upper thighs. As the hips finish extension, the athlete will quickly jump the feet out into the squat stance, placing them flat on the ground aggressively, while pulling down against the bar with the arms to move the body down. The elbows should be then whipped around the bar into the rack position as the athlete settles into a partial squat receiving position. The athlete should attempt to secure the elbows at full height in the rack position as the feet reconnect with the floor (the feet will reconnect first, but the effort to match them will help the turnover speed).

Note that the hips or thighs are not banging into the bar and bumping it away from the athlete. The athlete is using the lats to push the bar back into the body to create contact, and the hips move forward into the bar as they extend. If the bar is kept as close to the legs as possible prior to this, there cannot be a significant enough collision to cause the bar to bounce away from the body. Along the same lines, the contact of the bar and body is not itself part of the effort to elevate the bar—it's a consequence of ideal mechanics in this part of the lift.

With very light weights, e.g. the empty barbell, athletes will likely not extend the ankles considerably at the top of the pull because they will be already trying to get the feet back flat on the floor (this is demonstrated in the photos accompanying this section; the third photo is immediately after complete extension and the athlete is already starting to pull down). A natural degree of ankle extension at the top of the pull will begin to occur as the athlete moves onto great loading.

When the athlete is comfortable and consistent with performing the hang power clean with the empty bar, weight should be added incrementally. Small increases in weight will allow the athlete to progress to the ultimately appropriate weight for that time without changes in technique due to the mental—conscious or not—reaction to feeling large weight increases. At this point in the learning process, we want to find a weight that allows the athlete to perform the lift as accurately as possible—this requires a load greater than the empty bar, but caution should be taken to not exceed the weight that allows proper execution, even if it's presently very light. If the movement is practiced well, the athlete will progress quickly to heavier weights; if the weight is pushed prematurely, the athlete will simply deviate from proper technique and develop bad habits that will be difficult to correct later.

POWER CLEAN

Once the athlete is capable of the hang power clean, learning the power clean from the floor is simple (at least in principle) and generally quick. Athletes may be limited primarily by inflexibility when it comes to setting a proper starting position with the barbell on the floor. This can be addressed over time with flexibility work.

The most difficult part about moving an athlete from the hang to the floor is ensuring proper

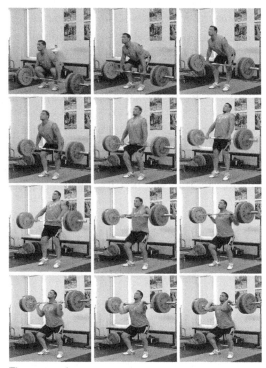
The power clean

positioning and timing going into the explosion phase. Athletes will typically try to begin the final acceleration effort too soon, and often will not maintain the proper posture and balance when moving from the floor to a position with the bar at the thighs. If the movement is taught well, these problems can usually be avoided fairly easily from the start. This progression is intended to help prevent this problem.

STEP 1 Starting Position

Our first step is teaching the athlete the proper starting position.
This will be the ideal position
for starting the lift, and it may
require modification for certain
athletes, such as those who are
very tall or inflexible.

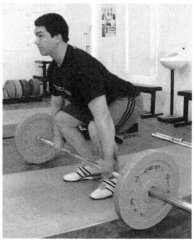

Clean starting position

The feet should be placed
with the heels approximately
under the hips or slightly wider with the toes turned out to
whatever degree is comfortable
for the athlete as long as it's not
excessive—usually this is about
5-15 degrees from the center-
line. The barbell should rest over the balls of the feet. The shins
do not need to be in contact with the bar, but they will be in close
proximity.

The athlete's arms should be oriented vertically when viewing
the athlete from the side. The leading edge of the shoulder will be
slightly in front of the bar with this vertical arm orientation. The
arms should be internally rotated to direct the points of the elbows
to the sides.

The back should be arched completely and tightly with the
head and eyes straight forward. The knees should be pushed out
to the sides slightly as space between the arms allows. The weight
should be balanced over the foot. It should not be dramatically
back over the heels with the bar still on the floor.

---

1 Starting Position

- Bar over balls of the feet
- Arms vertical
- Back arched tightly
- Knees out, points of elbows out and head up
- Weight balanced over the foot

STEP 2 Halting Clean Deadlift

The halting clean deadlift teaches the athlete how to move properly from the starting position into the position from which he or she will initiate the final explosion effort to accelerate the barbell upward. The pull from the floor to this point is primarily a positioning movement to set up the ideal position to explode from; it is not a direct effort to accelerate the bar itself, although it will begin to create upward momentum on the barbell. The key is teaching athletes right from the start that they will be more explosive if they are patient and time the lift correctly rather than attempting to accelerate directly off the floor.

The athlete should set the starting position and create tension against the bar momentarily before separating it from the floor. This will prevent unwanted shifts in balance and position when the bar breaks, as well as allow more force to be generated. Immediately as the bar separates, the athlete needs to shift the balance over the feet back to be slightly farther back toward the heels than the balls of the feet.

Moving slowly, the athlete will simply continue pushing with the legs to extend the knees, maintaining approximately the same back angle that was set in the starting position, actively keeping the bar as close to the legs as possible without dragging it. As the bar reaches the knees, the arms should still be vertical as they were in the start position.

Continuing to extend the knees, the athlete will stand until the bar is at the level of mid-thigh and stop. At this point, the

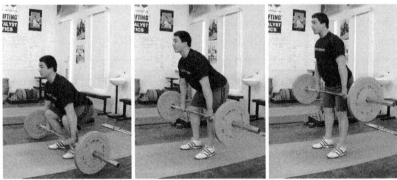

Halting clean deadlift: Start, mid-point, finish position.

knees will be only slightly bent, the shins vertical, and the bar will now be behind the shoulders slightly—the athlete needs to actively push the bar back in toward the body with the lats. Keeping the shoulders over the bar until this point is critical to generating explosiveness. They do not need to be very far forward of the bar, however.

After holding this mid-thigh position for 2-3 seconds, the athlete should return the barbell to the floor under control, attempting to reverse the movement as accurately as possible. Initially this drill should be done with light weights and 2-3 reps at a time. The athlete should feel tension in the hamstrings, glutes and back, particularly in the pause position at mid-thigh. This is not only teaching the athlete the proper movement and position, but strengthening the body for them.

Once the athlete can comfortably perform the halting clean deadlift, he or she is ready to power clean.

---

2 Halting Clean Deadlift

- Set the starting position tightly
- Separate the bar smoothly by pushing the legs through the floor and shift farther back toward the heels
- Maintain approximately the same back angle to keep the arms vertical until the bar passes the knees
- Extend the legs until the bar is at mid-thigh
- Stop and hold this position with the shoulders in front of the bar and the bar pushed back against the thighs

---

STEP 3 Power Clean

At this point the athlete can perform a power clean from the hang position and is able to lift the bar properly from the floor to the hang position. These two exercises simply need to be combined. Weights at this stage should be kept light enough that the athlete can perform the movement correctly without struggling.

Initially, the athlete should perform the power clean with a very slow lift from the floor to approximately mid-thigh. Without pausing here, the athlete will perform the power clean just as he or she did from the hang. This is simply a halting clean deadlift + hang power clean, but with no separation between the two. This slow pull to the hang position helps ensure that the athlete doesn't rush the explosion and provides more time to maintain proper balance and positioning. Generally 2-3 reps per set is advisable, although at this stage, rest between sets can be very brief.

When the athlete is able to demonstrate the exercise properly with this exaggeratedly slow first pull, the movement can be done at a more natural speed. However, it needs to be understood that the pull from the floor to the thigh will always be significantly slower than the explosion from the thighs up. As the athlete progresses to being able to power clean heavier weights, the effort during the first pull will become greater and greater, but the speed of the movement will remain comparatively slow because of the mechanics of the body in that position. Ultimately, the first pull

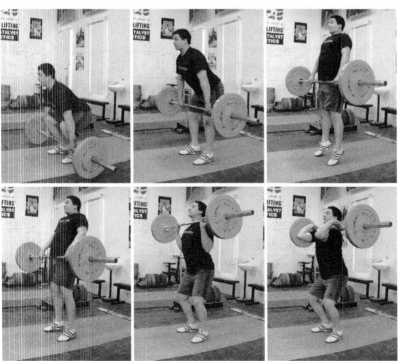

Power clean

can be as fast as the athlete can perform it without compromising proper positioning and timing.

Two ways to graduate the athlete's advancement to the actual power clean more slowly if necessary are using a two-position power clean or a segment power clean. The two-position power clean is simply a hang power clean followed immediately by a power clean. This complex allows the athlete to perform one rep from an easier, more comfortable position, then adds the pull from the floor, giving him or her the chance to focus on setting up to feel the same lift that was done from the hang.

The segment power clean is a power clean with a pause at the hang position. This is simply an exaggeration of the normal step— a slow pull to mid-thigh, a pause to ensure the position is perfect, then a hang power clean. This can be helpful for athletes who are struggling with keeping track of everything they're supposed to be doing. Once these are going well, the pause can be removed and the first pull to above the knee kept slow as needed.

---

3 Power Clean

- From a tight start position, lift the barbell slowly to mid-thigh
- As the bar nears mid-thigh, perform the power clean as practiced from the hang
- As consistency improves, the speed of the pull from the floor can be increased as long as it doesn't prevent proper positioning and timing

---

PUSH PRESS

With the ability to perform the power clean from the hang or floor, the athlete now has an excellent tool for hip and leg explosiveness. Before learning the more difficult power snatch, which will provide a similar training effect, the athlete can learn the jerk and its primary variations, including the push press, to provide some upper body explosive exercises, as well as exercises that emphasize the legs over the hips.

The push press is a valuable leg power and upper body strength exercise itself, but also a good step in the progression to learning the jerk.

STEP 1 Overhead Position

The first step in learning the push press is to establish the proper overhead position. This will ensure stability and safety for the shoulders, elbows and wrists. The overhead position for the push press will be the same for all press and jerk variations.

With the barbell placed behind the neck on top of the traps and a clean-width grip (half a fist to a fist-width outside the shoulders), the athlete will fully retract the shoulder blades and extend

---

1 Overhead Position
- Place the barbell directly above the base of the neck
- Forcefully retract the shoulder blades
- Keep the barbell in the palm

---

the upper back, maintaining tight abs. He or she will press the bar straight up, maintaining the forceful retraction of the shoulder blades. With the elbows fully extended, the barbell should be located directly over the base of the neck with the head pushed forward through the arms slightly.

The elbows should be fully extended and squeezed

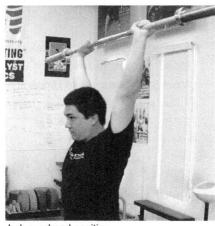
Jerk overhead position

tightly. The barbell should sit in the palms slightly behind the midline of the forearm and the grip should be as loose as possible while maintaining control of the bar.

STEP 2 Press

With the overhead position established, the lifter needs to learn the pressing mechanics of the push press (which will be the same for the punch down under the bar in the jerk). With the same grip on the bar used previously, the athlete will bring the bar to the shoulders, and keeping the upper back extended, push the shoulders forward and slightly up to create a shelf for the barbell. The bar should sit between the throat and the peak of the shoulders—pushing the shoulders forward will create a slight depression here that will allow the barbell to sit securely.

The athlete should keep the bar in the palms as much as possible rather than allowing it to move to the fingers

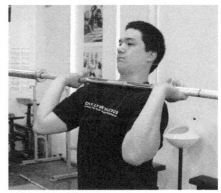
Jerk rack position

2 Press

- Start with the barbell in the jerk rack position
- Move the head back out of the way to press the bar up and back
- Move the elbows out and under the bar
- Finish securely in the proper overhead position

as it would in the rack position for the front squat and clean. The elbows should be spread to the sides and moved down while remaining at least slightly in front of the bar and the lats pushed out and up to help support the position. This position is very demanding of shoulder flexibility and may not be perfect for many athletes initially. The width of the grip can be adjusted in or out somewhat to see if the rack position can be improved.

From this jerk rack position, the athlete will push the bar up and slightly back, moving the head back out of the way as the bar passes. The bar cannot be pressed forward around the face. The elbows should be pushed out to the sides and moved under the bar as the bar leaves the shoulders rather than being left in front of the bar. As the barbell passes the head, it should continue moving back into place over the base of the neck and the head should move forward through the arms to establish the overhead position practiced previously.

From the rack position to the overhead position, the bar must move backward slightly—it needs to move in as direct a path as possible.

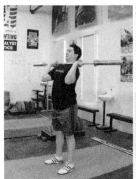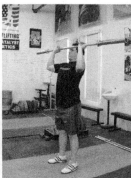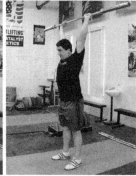

Press

STEP 3 Dip & Drive

The primary power element of the push press is the dip and drive of the legs to accelerate the barbell upward off the shoulders. Athletes need to understand from the start that this movement occurs entirely at the knees—there is no hinge of the hips.

The feet should be in the drive position— slightly wider than hip

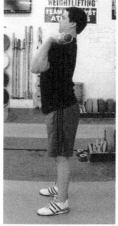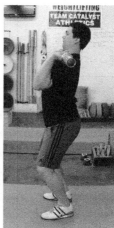

Dip position

width and the toes turned out slightly. With the barbell in the jerk rack position, the athlete will unlock the knees slightly and put tension on the quads, moving the weight to the heels while keeping the whole foot in contact with the floor. Maintaining this balance over the heels, the athlete will bend slowly only at the knees, keeping the torso vertical, dipping approximately 8-10% of his or her height (e.g. for a 6-foot tall athlete, the dip depth is approximately 5½ - 7 inches). The initiation of the dip must be smooth. At the bottom of the dip, an imaginary vertical line should pass through the end of the barbell, the hip and the ankle.

After reaching the bottom of the dip, the athlete will stand again slowly, maintaining the weight over the heels. If viewing the athlete from the side, the end of the barbell should move in a perfectly vertical line down and back up.

This slow and controlled dip should be practiced as much as

3 Dip & Drive
- Hold the barbell in the jerk rack position
- Stand with slightly unlocked knees and the weight over the heels
- Dip smoothly at the knees only approximately 8-10% of your height
- Stand again slowly, maintaining a vertical bar path

necessary for the athlete to be consistent with the proper positions and balance. Both are critical for successful jerks.

STEP 4 Push Press

The push press is now simply the combination of the dip, drive and press performed as one fluid movement. Athletes should keep in mind when performing the push press that it is powered primarily by the legs rather than the upper body. The legs accelerate the bar upward and the arms simply follow through to bring the bar into the overhead position.

The athlete will hold the bar in the jerk rack position with a loose grip, unlock the knees slightly and settle back over the heels. With a smooth bend of the knees, he or she will dip with a vertical torso and weight over the heels, then immediately change directions at the bottom and drive up powerfully with the legs, maintaining balance over the heels. With a forceful leg drive, the athlete will rise somewhat onto the balls of the feet; this is a sign of a proper drive and is not a problem as long as the athlete's weight remains back over the heel during this ankle extension.

The speed of

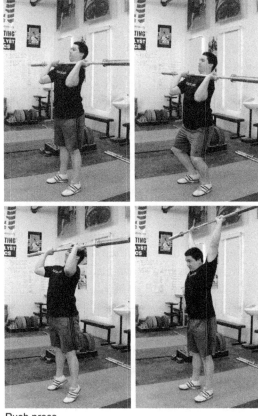

Push press

GREG EVERETT

the dip should never become so great that the shoulders drop out from under the bar—the bar must remain settled and connected tightly to the shoulders throughout the movement. With this restriction in mind, the dip can be as quick as possible to increase the elasticity of the movement.

As the bar leaves the shoulders, the athlete will keep the legs tight and straight and push the bar up and back with the arms aggressively. Just as in the press, the head must be pulled back to allow a direct path for the bar to move up and back over the base of the neck. The athlete should secure the overhead position tightly before returning the bar to the shoulders for subsequent reps.

Breath control and trunk pressurization are very important in the push press and jerk to prevent forward collapse of the upper back and forward shifting during the dip and drive.

---

4 Push Press

- Start with the barbell in the jerk rack position and weight on the heels
- Dip smoothly at the knees only
- Immediately change directions at the bottom of the dip and drive up forcefully with the legs
- As the bar leaves the shoulders, push up and back aggressively with the arms
- Secure the bar in the proper overhead position

POWER JERK

The athlete is now familiar with the movement of the dip and drive that accelerates the barbell upward, and the mechanics of the arms to continue pushing the barbell up into the overhead position, which will be the same used to push the athlete down under the bar into the receiving position for the jerk. The next step is to learn the simplest jerk variant—the power jerk.

STEP 1 Tall Power Jerk

The first step is learning to push down under the barbell. Just as in the clean, the athlete will use the arms to move his or her body down under the bar after using the lower body to accelerate it upward.

The athlete will stand with the feet in the drive position used for the push press and the barbell in the jerk rack position, then press the barbell halfway up to approximately the level of the forehead. The head should be pulled back out of the way and the elbows moved out to the sides and approximately under the bar.

---

1 Tall Power Jerk
- Start with the barbell pressed to forehead level
- Jump the feet quickly to the squat position
- Punch down against the bar
- Land in a quarter squat with the bar locked out in the overhead position

---

　　　　　　　　　　　　　　　　　　　GREG EVERETT

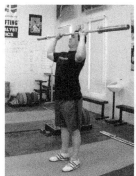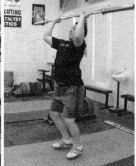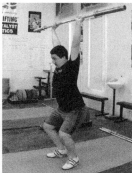

Tall power jerk

This is the starting position for the drill.

From this partial press starting position, the athlete will quickly jump the feet out into the squat position, landing flat-footed, while punching aggressively with the arms against the bar to push the body down into a quarter squat. The athlete should land in the quarter squat with the elbows locked tightly in extension. This receiving position should be held momentarily to ensure stability before standing.

STEP 2 Power Jerk

The athlete needs now to simply combine the dip and drive of the push press to accelerate the bar upward with the punch down against the bar of the tall power jerk to move down into the receiving position.

With the feet in the drive position, weight on the heels, and the barbell in the jerk rack position, the athlete will dip smoothly at

2 Power Jerk
- Dip and drive just as in the push press
- When the leg drive is complete, jump the feet to the squat position
- As the feet are moving, punch down against the bar
- Land in a quarter squat with the elbows locked in the correct overhead position

the knees, then drive against the floor aggressively, making sure the trunk remains vertical. As the bar leaves the shoulders, the athlete will quickly jump the feet out into the squat stance while pushing down against the bar with the arms. Just as in the push press, the head needs to be moved back out of the way and the push with the arms directed slightly backward to locate the barbell over the base of the neck. The athlete should finish in a quarter squat with the elbows locked tightly in the correct overhead position. The athlete should aim to lock the elbows out overhead at the same time the feet reconnect with the floor. Just as with the rack in the power clean, the feet will land first, but the effort to time the lift this way will encourage better speed and aggression.

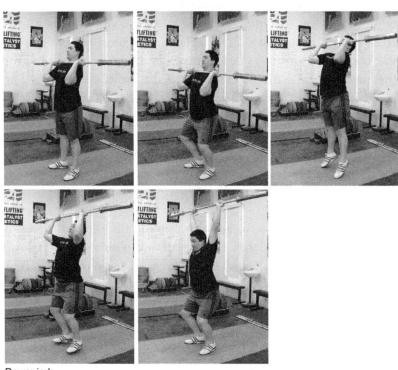

Power jerk

SPLIT JERK

The split jerk is the final jerk variation to learn. It allows deeper receiving positions with much less demand on shoulder mobility than the power jerk, as well as greater stability. The split foot position also offers some footwork, balance and hip and ankle stability to the athlete's training. It's recommended that athletes learn to split with both

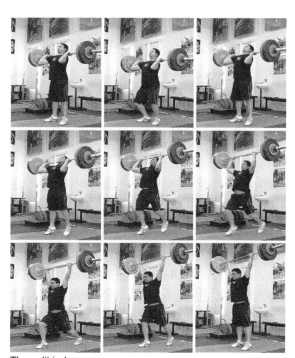

The split jerk

feet forward and to alternate split legs in training to maintain balanced flexibility and strength in the legs and hips. Athletes who tend to use a staggered stance with the same foot forward primarily (e.g. striking and throwing athletes) can use their normal lead leg more than the other as long mobility and strength disparities are avoided in other manners[1].

---

1 Thanks to Mike Gattone for this idea

STEP 1 Split Footwork

A proper split po-
sition is necessary
both for optimizing
performance and
maximizing safety
in the jerk. If want-
ing to find the ath-
lete's natural lead
leg, perform a set
of walking lunges—
the leg with which

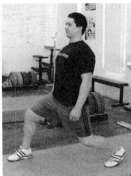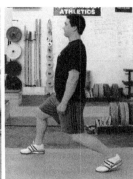

Split position

the athlete naturally steps forward with first will nearly invariably
be the leg he or she will be strongest leading with in the split jerk.

The athlete will step into a lunge position with the chosen lead
leg, keeping the width of the feet at least the same as in the squat
stance. Placing the feet in line with each other or nearly so greatly
reduces the lateral stability of the split position. The length and
depth of the split should be adjusted until the front shin is vertical
and the front thigh is approximately 20-40 degrees relative to the
floor.

The rear knee must be bent at least slightly and the rear heel
elevated. The athlete needs to keep the balls of the rear foot in
contact with the floor—he or she should be up on the toes only.
Weight should be evenly balanced between the feet—most athletes
will naturally place much more weight on the front foot.

The front foot should point straight forward or very slightly

---

1 Split Footwork

- Front foot flat, pointed forward, weight on heel, front shin vertical
- Front thigh 20-40 degrees relative to the floor
- Rear heel elevated, foot turned in slightly, weight on balls of the foot
- Width of feet at least the same as the squat stance
- Rear knee bent and spine in neutral position
- Weight balanced evenly between front and back feet

GREG EVERETT

inward. The heel of the rear foot should be turned out somewhat to keep the foot aligned with the leg. The spine should be neutral and the hips under the shoulders. If the lower back is hyperextended in this position, the athlete is most likely not bending the back knee enough.

When the athlete has learned the correct split position, he or she can drill the movement from the drive position to the split. Standing in the drive position, making sure the weight is over the heels, the athlete will jump the feet into the split position, making sure his or her weight is balanced evenly between the two feet and the hips are under the shoulders. The rear foot should stay very close to the floor as it moves back, and the front foot should be picked up enough to reconnect it flat against the floor in the proper position.

STEP 2 Split Jerk

The athlete now has all the tools necessary to perform the split jerk. However, this lift can be challenging for many because of the introduction of the horizontal foot movement to what was previously confined to a vertical movement. Athletes should understand from the start that the dip and drive of the split jerk is identical to the push press and power jerk—it must remain vertical. Only after this vertical dip and drive is completed do the feet split.

The athlete will begin with the feet in the drive position and the barbell in the jerk rack position, the weight back on the heels, and the trunk pressurized and tight. He or she will dip smoothly and drive straight up aggressively, moving the head back out of

---

2 Split Jerk

- Dip and drive just as in the push press and power jerk
- When the leg drive is complete, jump the feet to the split position
- As the feet are moving, punch down against the bar
- Land in a balanced split position with the elbows locked in the correct overhead position

---

the way and attempting to push the bar slightly back. As the drive is completed and the bar leaves the shoulders, the athlete will split the feet quickly and punch down against the bar to receive the lift with locked elbows in a balanced split position.

After stabilizing the position, the athlete will step back approximately a third of the way with the front foot, then step forward the rest of the way with the rear foot. This method of recovering to a standing position minimizes bar movement and maximizes stability.

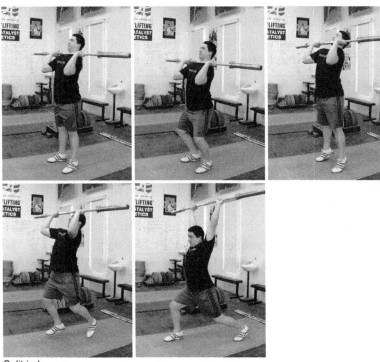

Split jerk

GREG EVERETT

HANG POWER SNATCH

With the ability to perform the power clean and the jerk, the athlete now has two tools for explosive training; one that emphasizes the knees and hips together, and one that emphasizes the knees and upper body. The power snatch, first from the hang and then from the floor, will provide another tool to the set that, similar to the power clean, involves both the knees and hips, but is even faster and also involves the element of overhead strength and stability.

The power snatch is often taught to athletes with a narrow grip. In some cases, there is good reason for this. However, here the athlete is encouraged to use the wide grip used by weightlifters for the snatch. For our purposes, this wide grip allows the bar to move into the hips rather than the thighs, which will allow the athlete to be more explosive and to extend the hips more completely; additionally, it will allow a better position overhead due to the reduced demand on mobility.

It should become obvious quickly that the teaching progression for the power snatch is essentially the same as it was for the power clean. The lifts are fundamentally identical, with the exception of the receiving positions and grip width. This has some slight effect on the mechanics, but in principle, the lifts are no different: the legs and hips accelerate the barbell upward, and the arms pull the lifter down under the bar.

STEP 1 Overhead Position

Our first step is learning the proper overhead position in which to receive the power snatch. To find the grip width, the athlete will hold the bar at arms' length and adjust until the bar contacts the body in the crease of the hips. This will be the default grip width; adjustments to account for unusual body proportions or to work around injury or discomfort can be made subsequently.

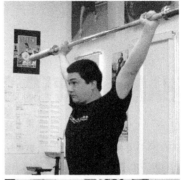

With this snatch grip, the athlete will bring the bar to the back of the neck, tightly retract the shoulder blades, and press the bar straight up. The overhead position of the snatch is identical to that of the jerk other than the width of the grip. The shoulder blades will be fully retracted and somewhat up-

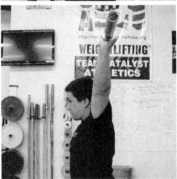

Snatch overhead position

wardly rotated; the elbows will be extended forcefully and oriented approximately halfway between back and to the sides; the trunk will be inclined forward slightly, the head pushed through the arms, and the barbell directly over the base of the neck; the bar will be in the palms slightly behind the midline of the forearm and the grip as relaxed as possible while maintaining control of the bar.

---

1 Overhead Position

- Use a grip width that places the bar in the crease of the hips when at arms' length
- Place the barbell directly above the base of the neck
- Forcefully retract the shoulder blades
- Keep the barbell in the palm with a relaxed grip

STEP 2 Hang Position

The hang start position for the power snatch is identical to that of the power clean. With the snatch grip on the barbell, the athlete will set the back tightly, hinge at the hips, unlocking the knees and sliding the bar down the thigh until it stops just above the kneecaps. The feet should be in the pulling position—approximately hip width or slightly wider with the toes turned out somewhat.

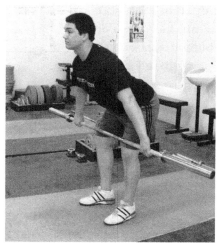
Snatch hang position

In this position, the shins and arms should be approximately vertical, the back arched tightly with the head and eyes straight forward, the points of the elbows turned to the sides (upper arm internally rotated), and the weight somewhat behind mid-foot (more pressure on the heels than on the balls of the feet, but still full foot contact with the floor). As part of the effort to maintain a proper back arch, the lats should be engaged, and this will help push the barbell back toward the body as the athlete extends.

---

2 Hang Position

- Feet hip width and toes turned out slightly
- Shins and arms approximately vertical
- Bar just above knee
- Weight toward heels
- Back arched and head forward

STEP 3 Jump & Bump

Just as in the power clean, the "jump & bump" is the explosion phase of the power snatch: the violent extension of the knees and hips to accelerate the barbell upward.

Before adding speed to this drill,

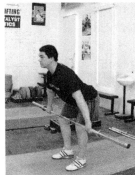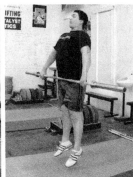

Jump & bump

the athlete will first do a slow movement to feel the proper positions. Starting in the hang position, the athlete will start by pushing against the floor with the legs, keeping the barbell as close to the thighs as possible without contacting them. When the bar reaches the upper-thigh, the athlete will extend the hips as the knees continue extending. The bar should come into contact with the crease of the hips as the athlete completes the combined hip and knee extension through the active push back of the bar into the body with the lats. In this final extended position, the athlete's weight should be more on the heels than the balls of the feet, the bar touching the crease of the hips at arms' length, the points of the elbows still turned to the sides, the knees straight and the hips slightly hyperextended, placing the shoulders slightly behind the hips. Again, it's important to ensure that this hyperextension is actually occurring at the hip, not in the lumbar spine, through activation of the glutes.

When this basic movement is done properly, the athlete will move on to the full-speed drill. From the hang starting position,

---

3 Jump & Bump

- Start in the hang position
- Push against the floor with the legs
- Jump and extend the hips completely
- Push the bar back into the hips

GREG EVERETT

the athlete will initiate the movement with the same push of the legs against the floor, then jump as the bar reaches upper thigh level, extending the hips completely while pushing the bar back into the hips with the lats. The goal is not to do a maximal vertical jump, but to feel the simultaneous explosion of knees and hips with proper contact of the bar against the body.

During this movement, the athlete's arms should remain as relaxed as possible, being extended only by the weight of the barbell pulling on them. As the jump is completed, the bar should be kept in tight against the body, not allowed to bounce off the hips and swing forward. The athlete's feet should be landing on the floor in the same place they started; moving forward or backward indicates that the athlete's balance is starting or shifting too far in the direction of movement.

STEP 4 Pull

The pull drill is the same for the power snatch as it was for the power clean. The wider hand placement will typically make athletes feel weaker in the movement, and they must be careful to not swing the bar forward away from the body. Again, this movement is the acceleration of the athlete's body down under the bar.

Standing tall with the feet in the pulling position, the athlete will make sure the points of the elbows are turned to the sides and the weight is more on the heels than the balls of the feet. Simul-

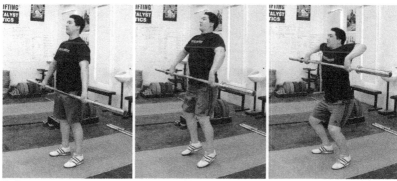

Pull

┌───┐
│ **4 Pull**   │
│   │
│ • Start standing tall with feet in the pulling position │
│ • Pull down against the bar with the arms   │
│ • Move the feet to the squat position and sit into a partial squat │
│ • Elbows move up and to the sides with the bar close to the body │
└───┘

taneously, the athlete will pull down against the bar with the arms and jump the feet out into the squat position, squatting partially down with the effort to pull against the bar. The elbows should move up and out to the sides, keeping the barbell and body in immediate proximity to each other.

The movement of the feet should be quick and aggressive, with as little elevation as possible, and the feet should reconnect with the floor flat.

STEP 5 Punch

In the punch drill, the athlete will learn to finish the pull under the power snatch properly, which actually means a push against the bar. With a snatch grip, the athlete will bring the bar to the back of the neck just as he or she did when first learning the overhead position. The feet should be in the pulling position and the weight more on the heels than the balls of the feet.

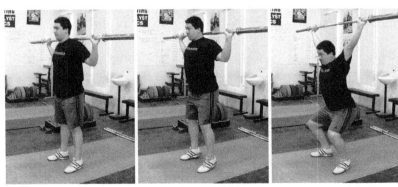

Punch

5 Punch

- Start with the feet in the pulling position and the bar behind the neck
- Jump the feet to the squat position
- Punch down against the bar into quarter squat depth
- Lock the elbows as the feet reconnect with the floor

Just as in the previous drill, the athlete will perform a jump of the feet out into the squat stance while moving down into a quarter squat, but now this movement will be accompanied by an aggressive punch against the bar with the arms. The goal is to lock out the elbows completely and forcefully at the same time the feet reconnect flat with the floor with the athlete at quarter squat depth. The athlete should ensure the proper overhead position and balance over the feet before standing.

STEP 6 Hang Power Snatch

The athlete can now put the previous drills together into a hang power snatch: Jump & bump, pull & punch. Initially the movement should be practiced with an empty barbell as the previous drills were.

Starting in the hang position, the athlete will first push against the floor with the legs. As the bar reaches mid to upper-thigh, he or she will extend the hips explosively while continuing to punch the legs into the floor, using the lats to push the bar back into the hips.

6 Hang Power Snatch

- Start in the hang position
- Push against the floor with the legs
- Extend the hips explosively with continued leg drive
- Push the bar back into the hips with the lats
- Move the feet out to the squat position and reconnect flat
- Pull down against the bar with the elbows high and to the sides
- Punch the arms up against the bar and secure the overhead position

As the athlete finishes the extension, he or she will aggressively pull down with the arms against the bar, keeping the elbows to the sides, turn the bar over and punch it straight up over the back of the neck while jumping the feet quickly into the squat position and reconnecting them flat.

When the athlete is comfortable and consistent with performing the hang power snatch with the empty bar, weight should be added incrementally. Small increases in weight will allow the athlete to progress to the ultimately appropriate weight for that time without changes in technique due to the mental—conscious or not—reaction to feeling large weight increases. At this point in the learning process, we want to find a weight that allows the athlete to perform the lift as accurately as possible—this usually requires a load greater than the empty bar, but caution should be taken to not exceed the weight that allows proper execution, even if it's presently very light. If the movement is practiced well, the athlete will progress quickly to heavier weights; if the weight is pushed

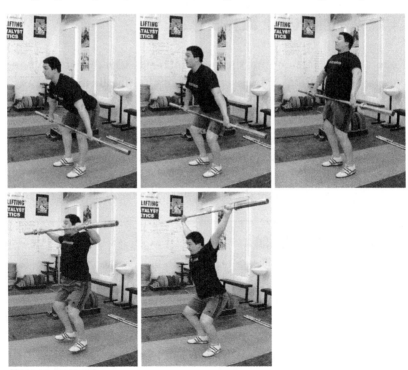

Hang power snatch

prematurely, the athlete will simply deviate from proper technique and develop bad habits that will be difficult to correct later.

With the hang power snatch, it's important that the athlete not be allowed to use more weight than can be locked out securely and properly. If the athlete receives the bar overhead with bent elbows, bends the back or otherwise finds ways to squeeze in under the bar rather than lifting it and pulling under properly, the point of the exercise is being defeated and the athlete is exposing him- or herself to injury.

POWER SNATCH

Once the athlete is capable of the hang power snatch, learning the power snatch from the floor is simple, although flexibility may become a problem in the starting position even more so than with the power clean. This can be addressed over time with flexibility work. The lift can be performed from below the knee from blocks or the hang in the meantime.

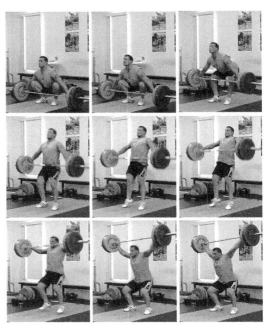

The power snatch

STEP 1 Starting Position

Our first step is teaching the athlete the proper starting position. This will be the ideal position for starting the lift, and it may require modification for certain athletes, such as those who are very tall or inflexible. The snatch starting position, because of the wide grip, is even more demanding of flexibility and less forgiving of long legs than the power clean starting position.

The feet should be placed in the pulling position—the heels approximately under the hips or slightly wider with the toes turned out to whatever degree is comfortable for the athlete as long as it's not excessive—usually this is about 5-15 degrees from the centerline. The barbell should rest over the balls of the feet. The shins do not need to be in contact with the bar, but they will be in close proximity.

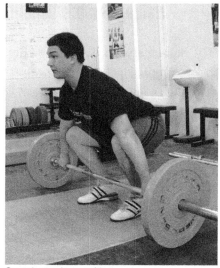

Snatch starting position

The athlete's arms should be oriented vertically when viewing the athlete from the side. The leading edge of the shoulder will be slightly in front of the bar with this vertical arm orientation. The arms should be internally rotated to direct the points of the elbows to the sides.

The back should be arched completely and tightly with the head and eyes straight forward. The knees should be pushed out to the sides slightly as space between the arms allows. This outward flaring of the knees is critical to allow the athlete to get into such a deep starting position. The weight should be balanced over the foot. It should not be dramatically back over the heels.

---

1 Starting Position

- Bar over balls of the feet
- Arms vertical
- Back arched tightly
- Knees out, elbows out and head up

STEP 2 Halting Snatch Deadlift

The halting snatch deadlift teaches the athlete how to move prop-erly from the starting position into the position from which he or she will initiate the final explosion effort to accelerate the barbell upward. The pull from the floor to this point is primarily a posi-tioning movement to set up the ideal position to explode from; it is not a direct effort to accelerate the bar itself, although it will begin to create upward momentum on the barbell. Athletes need to understand right away that they will be more explosive if they are patient and time the lift correctly rather than attempting to ac-celerate directly off the floor.

The athlete should set the starting position and create tension against the bar momentarily before separating it from the floor. This will prevent unwanted shifts in balance and position when the bar breaks, as well as allow more force to be generated. Imme-diately as the bar separates, the athlete needs to shift the balance over the feet back to be slightly farther back toward the heels than the balls of the feet.

Moving slowly, the athlete will simply continue pushing with the legs to extend the knees, maintaining approximately the same back angle that was set in the starting position, actively keeping the bar as close to the legs as possible without dragging it. As the bar reaches the knees, the arms should still be vertical and the shoul-ders directly above the bar as they were in the start position.

Continuing to extend the knees, the athlete will stand until the bar is at the level of the upper-thigh and stop. At this point, the

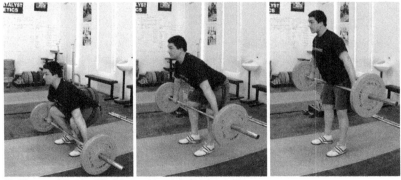

Halting snatch deadlift: Start, mid-point, finish position

GREG EVERETT

knees will be only slightly bent, the shins vertical, and the bar will now be behind the shoulders slightly—the athlete needs to actively push the bar back in toward the body with the lats. Keeping the shoulders over the bar until this point is critical to generating explosiveness. They do not need to be very far forward of the bar, however.

After holding this upper-thigh position for 2-3 seconds, the athlete should return the barbell to the floor under control, attempting to reverse the movement as accurately as possible. Initially this drill should be done with light weights and 2-3 reps at a time. The athlete should feel tension in the hamstrings, glutes and back, particularly in the pause position at upper-thigh. This is not only teaching the athlete the proper movement and position, but strengthening the body for them.

Once the athlete can comfortably perform the halting snatch deadlift, he or she is ready to power snatch.

---

2 Halting Snatch Deadlift

- Set the starting position tightly
- Separate the bar smoothly by pushing the legs through the floor and shift farther back toward the heels
- Maintain approximately the same back angle to keep the arms vertical until the bar passes the knees
- Extend the legs until the bar is at upper-thigh
- Stop and hold this position with the shoulders in front of the bar and the bar pushed back against the thighs

---

STEP 3 Power Snatch

At this point the athlete can perform a power snatch from the hang position and is able to lift the bar properly from the floor to the hang position. These two exercises simply need to be combined. Weights at this stage should be kept light enough that the athlete can perform the movement correctly without struggling.

Initially, the athlete should perform the power snatch with a

3 Power Snatch

- From a tight start position, slowly lift the barbell to mid-thigh
- As the bar reaches the mid-thigh, perform the power snatch as practiced from the hang
- As consistency improves, the speed of the pull from the floor can be increased as long as it doesn't prevent proper positioning and timing

very slow lift from the floor to mid-thigh. Without pausing here, the athlete will perform the power snatch just as he or she did from the hang. This is simply a halting snatch deadlift + hang power snatch, but with no separation between the two. This slow pull to the hang position helps ensure that the athlete doesn't rush the explosion and provides more time to maintain proper balance and positioning. Generally 2-3 reps per set is advisable, although at this stage, rest between sets can be very brief.

When the athlete is able to demonstrate the exercise properly with this exaggeratedly slow first pull, the movement can be done at a more natural speed. However, it needs to be understood that the pull from the floor to mid-thigh will always be significantly slower than the explosion from mid-thigh up. As the athlete progresses to being able to power snatch heavier weights, the effort during the first pull will become greater and greater, but the speed of the movement will remain comparatively slow because of the mechanics of the body in that position. Ultimately, the first pull can be as fast as the athlete can perform it without compromising proper positioning and timing.

Two ways to slow the athlete's advancement to the actual power snatch if necessary are using a two-position power snatch or a segment power snatch. The two-position power snatch is simply a hang power snatch followed immediately by a power snatch. This complex allows the athlete to perform one rep from an easier, more comfortable position, then adds the pull from the floor, giving him or her the chance to focus on setting up to feel the same lift that was done from the hang.

The segment power snatch is a power snatch with a pause at the hang position. This is simply an exaggeration of the normal step—a slow pull to mid-thigh, a pause to ensure the position is perfect, then a hang power snatch. This can be helpful for athletes who are struggling with keeping track of everything they're supposed to be doing. Once these are going well, the pause can be removed and the first pull to above the knee kept slow as needed.

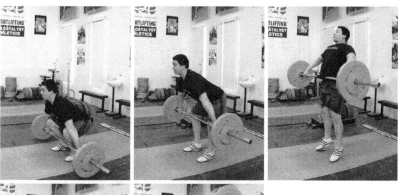

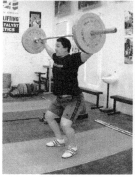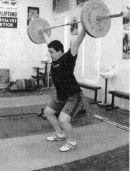

Power snatch

CLEAN

The clean and snatch are the final Olympic lifts for the athlete to learn. These are the complete competition lifts (the clean is always followed by a jerk in competition) and will offer athletes more training options. However, these lifts also require a significant degree of specific mobility that many athletes will not currently possess or wish to

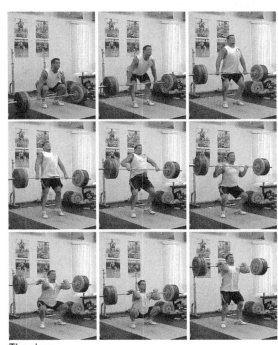

The clean

invest the time and energy to develop. For ambitious athletes who are not presently flexible enough to safely perform the lifts but wish to do so, this book includes information on developing the requisite mobility in the flexibility chapter.

The athlete is already familiar with the mechanics of the clean from learning and practicing the power clean. Fortunately the two lifts are identical, if properly performed, with the exception of the ultimate squat depth during the receipt of the barbell. Learning the clean now will be more a process of strengthening the front squat and building confidence in receiving heavy weights in lower positions.

STEP 1 Front Squat

The first step in progressing to the clean is learning the front squat. The athlete has already learned the rack position for the barbell during the power clean progression. With the bar in the clean rack position, the athlete will place the feet slightly wider than hip width with the toes turned out to whatever degree is comfortable, usually approximately 15-30 degrees from the centerline.

After pressurizing and stabilizing the trunk, the athlete will squat slowly, bending the knees and hips simultaneously and maintaining an upright posture. It's important that the athlete not break and lead with the hips before the knees—this will encourage forward leaning, which greatly limits the athlete's ability to support the weight. The knees should track over the toes to keep each thigh parallel with the corresponding foot.

In the bottom position, the knee joint should be closed as much as is possible while maintaining the correct extension of the lower back. The more flexible the athlete's hips and ankles are, the lower this will be. If an athlete cannot sit into a sound front squat to at least a depth below parallel, it's recommended that use of the clean be postponed until flexibility can be improved further.

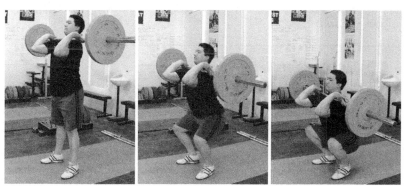

Front squat

The athlete's weight should remain balanced across the foot with a slight preference for the heel. When standing from the bottom of the squat, the athlete should lead with the elbows and chest, forcing the maintenance of the upright trunk.

---

1 Front Squat

- Hold the barbell in the clean rack position
- Pressurize the trunk and lock the spine in proper extension
- Bend at the knees and hips together
- Maintain balance slightly behind mid-foot
- Recover by leading with the elbows and chest

STEP 2 Power Clean + Front Squat

When the athlete is comfortable with the front squat, we can move on to the clean in at least a rudimentary form. The athlete will simply perform a power clean, hold the receiving position momentarily and make any adjustments necessary, such as correcting improperly positioned feet, then front squat from that position. Athletes can also start from the hang to simplify this first step. This is a better option if lifting from the floor is creating too many distractions for the athlete and the power clean is not being executed well.

The upward explosion of the lift should be reduced slightly in intensity to allow the athlete a chance to focus on pulling lower under the bar.

---

2 Power Clean + Front Squat

- Power clean (from floor or hang)
- Reduce upward explosion intensity and emphasize the pull down
- Hold and adjust receiving position as needed
- Front squat from the receiving position

GREG EVERETT

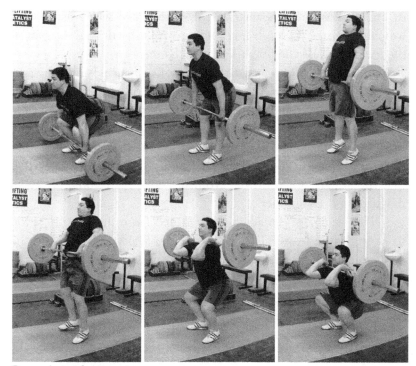

Power clean + front squat

STEP 3 Clean

Finally, the athlete will simply remove the pause from the previous step. The execution of the lift should remain the same in essence. As the athlete meets the bar with the shoulders, he or she will smoothly squat to the bottom. Athletes should reduce the force

3 Clean

- Perform the same pull used in the power clean
- Pull down under the bar with the arms after exploding with the legs and hips
- Sit into a squat as you pull down and spin the elbows around the bar
- Recover from the squat leading with the elbows and chest

of the explosion somewhat in this early stage when using light weights to force themselves to pull down under the bar. However, the mechanics of the lift should not change.

The lighter the weight, the higher of a squat position the athlete will be in when the bar reaches the rack position on the shoulders; as the weight increases, so will the depth of the squat at the point the bar is racked. The athlete needs to practice meeting the bar with the shoulders at whatever height the barbell is elevated to and immediately and smoothly sitting into the squat. It's important that the athlete not drop out from under the bar and let it crash down onto the shoulders.

The clean can initially be performed from the hang position to simplify the movement and allow the athlete to focus on the new element of squatting under. A complex of 1 hang clean + 1 clean can be performed to help then transition to the clean.

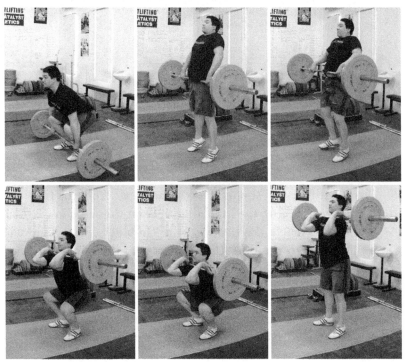

Clean

GREG EVERETT

SNATCH

The snatch is the final lift in the progression for two simple reasons: it's the most technically complex, and possibly more important, it demands the most flexibility of any of the lifts. Because of this, the snatch may be inaccessible to many athletes. It does offer unique training benefits, but for many athletes, those benefits are not worth the time

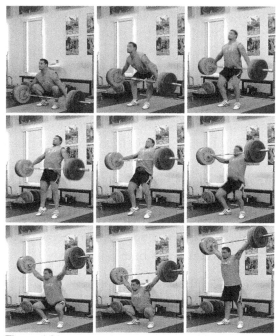

The snatch

and energy necessary to prepare themselves in terms of mobility to perform the lift properly and safely.

STEP 1 Overhead Squat

The athlete will need to first learn to overhead squat to full depth (as well as demonstrate the mobility to do so) before learning to

1 Overhead Squat

- Push press the barbell into the proper overhead position from behind the neck
- Squat slowly with upright posture and tight upper back
- Recover by pushing up against the bar and following it with the body

snatch. With the same grip used for the power snatch and the barbell behind the neck, the athlete will push press the bar into the overhead position learned for the power snatch. Ensuring the feet are in the proper squat stance, he or she will squat slowly to the bottom, maintaining an upright trunk, continuing to retract the shoulder blades tightly, and pushing the barbell straight up over the base of the neck. The stability and consistency of the overhead position is critical.

From the bottom of the squat, the athlete will recover by pushing up against the barbell and following it with the body. This will help keep the barbell positioned properly as well as help prevent the athlete from leading with the hips and tipping forward as he or she stands.

If the athlete is unable to sit into an overhead squat to a depth at least below parallel with the bar in the proper overhead position and the feet flat and balanced, it's recommended that snatching be postponed until flexibility is improved.

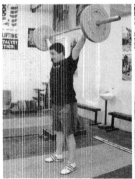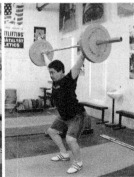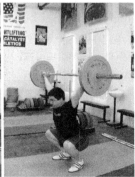

Overhead squat

GREG EVERETT

STEP 2 Power Snatch + Overhead Squat

The initial snatch will simply be a combination of a power snatch and an overhead squat. The athlete can begin with a hang power snatch if needed to simplify.

Following the power snatch, the athlete will hold the partial squat receiving position and make any adjustments, for example to the squat stance, then squat into the bottom position directly. As the athlete practices, the consistency of the receiving position will improve and less adjustment will be necessary.

2 Power Snatch + Overhead Squat

- Power snatch (from the hang or floor)
- Reduce upward explosion intensity and emphasize the pull down
- Hold and adjust receiving position as needed
- Overhead squat from the receiving position

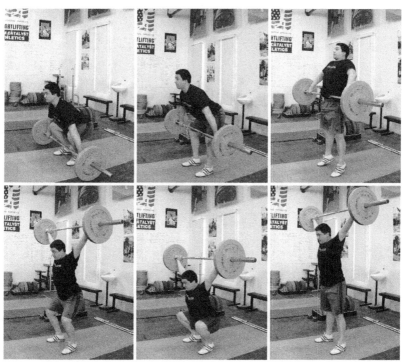

Power snatch + overhead squat

The upward explosion of the lift should be reduced slightly in intensity to allow the athlete a chance to focus on pulling lower under the bar.

STEP 3 Snatch

Finally, the athlete will perform the snatch by pulling down under the bar farther and squatting immediately as part of the same movement rather than a subsequent action.

Athletes will typically do better starting from the hang, as this not only reduces the elements they need to think about, but will allow them to elevate the barbell less, which will force them to be more aggressive pulling down under the bar into a lower receiving position.

Just like in the clean, when first starting and working with light weights, athletes will need to reduce the power of the upward

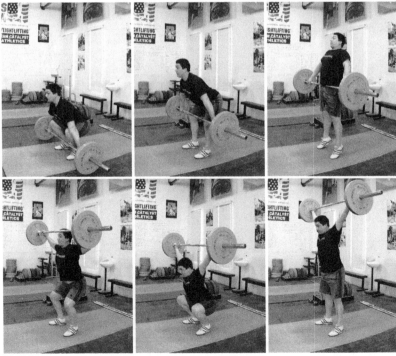

Snatch

explosion somewhat and focus on pulling down into a deeper receiving position.

Athletes need to be patient with the snatch and wait until the bar is around the upper thigh to initiate the explosive acceleration effort. It will be common for athletes to attempt to accelerate too early, and even to rush the lift directly off the floor. Performing the snatch initially with a 2-3 second count from the floor to upper thigh prior to the final upward explosion will help athletes time the movement properly.

---

3 Snatch

- Perform the pull of the power snatch
- Pull down under the bar with the arms after exploding with the legs and hips
- Sit into a squat as you pull down and punch up against the bar
- Recover from the squat leading with the bar

LOWERING THE BARBELL

When performing multiple-rep sets of the Olympic lifts, often the most difficult part is lowering the bar between reps. For lifts that begin from the floor, this is not an issue as the bar can be dropped onto the platform. For lifts that begin in the hang or for consecutive reps in the jerk, the bar must be lowered under control. There are ways to do this safely and relatively comfortably that all athletes should practice—the only thing worse than getting hurt doing a lift is getting hurt between lifts.

Snatch & Clean

When lowering the bar from overhead after a snatch, the athlete will begin by slowly bending the arms under control to bring the bar down as low as can be managed in this position. At this point, he or she will quickly flip the elbows from under to over the bar, keeping it as close to the body as possible. The clean will begin with this flipping of the elbows from under to over the bar. As the elbows flip over, he or she will pop up onto the toes or jump slight-

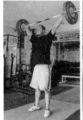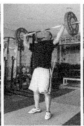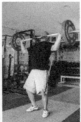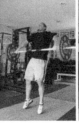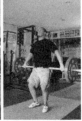

Lowering the snatch or power snatch

GREG EVERETT

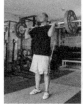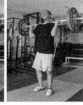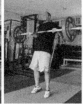

Lowering the clean or power clean

ly to meet the bar with the thighs, absorbing the force by dropping back to the heels and bending the knees. The thighs will also create somewhat of a shelf to catch the weight and reduce the strain on the grip. From here, the weight can be lowered in the same manner as a deadlift. To further reduce the height from which the bar must drop, the athlete may choose to dip slightly at the knees while bending the elbows prior to jumping up to meet the bar.

In some cases of multiple-rep snatches from the floor when using straps, the lifter may choose to lower the bar before standing until the final rep. This can be done by, from the bottom of the squat, guiding the bar forward and down as the athlete begins standing in order to bring the hips and bar together. From this point, the rest of the movement is like lowering the bar from overhead; that is, the athlete will absorb the bar with a bend of the knees, and then drop the bar to the floor under control.

Jerk

With the jerk, the bar will be brought back to the rack position on the shoulders by the athlete first lowering it by bending the arms, then popping up onto the toes to bring the shoulders up to meet the falling bar, and absorbing the load by dropping to the heels and bending the knees as he or she would when lowering a snatch or clean, keeping the torso upright. From here the bar can be lowered to the floor as the clean is, or it can be replaced in a rack.

Overhead lifts can also be lowered to the shoulders behind the neck. This will be most common with snatch push presses or snatch balances, but may also be the preferred location for athletes after finishing a set of jerks, push presses or presses. The process

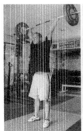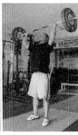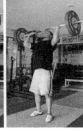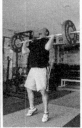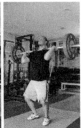

Lowering the jerk or push press

is the same as for bringing the bar down in the front—the athlete simply needs to keep the head out of the way, keep the shoulders shrugged up to ensure a muscular landing pad rather than a bony one, and to prevent dropping the chest as the weight of the bar is absorbed.

Dropping the Bar

Dropping the bar after a successful lift should not be a careless action. The lifter should maintain contact with the bar until it passes his or her waist, guiding it down safely away from him- or herself. This practice is an effort to maintain safety for both the lifter and the other athletes nearby. Different types of bumper plates will bounce to varying heights when dropped—some quite high, particularly in combination with the springier rubber tiles of some platforms—so the lifter should be careful to continue watching the bar as it drops and bounces and to keep his or her hands clear to avoid jamming fingers or a wrist against a rebounding bar. It's important as well to make sure the platform is clear of any spare plates off of which the bar could bounce in an unexpected direction and collide with the athlete or another nearby. Along the same lines, before the athlete drops the bar, he or she should make sure no other lifter has wandered into the area and inadvertently placed him or herself in the path of the bar.

PROGRAM DESIGN

Once the chosen Olympic lifts or variants have been learned by the athlete, they can be used in training. The first priority for all athletic training is safety. With regard to the Olympic lifts specifically, the coach and athlete must be diligent in avoiding strain or injury to the wrists, elbows, shoulders and knees in particular. Nothing about the Olympic lifts is inherently dangerous; but improper execution or programming, or the inadequate preparation of athletes, creates opportunity for injury.

In the context of athletic training, the goal of using the Olympic lifts is to develop athletic traits such as power and strength; the amount of weight actually lifted is essentially incidental. This does not mean that the weight used in the lifts is irrelevant—just as with any other exercise, the loading used will influence the training effect. The point that must be kept in mind at all times by the coach and athlete, both when designing programs and training, is that the quality of the movement is always a priority over the amount of weight moved. By maintaining this perspective, the athlete will benefit as much as possible from the use of the lifts while avoiding situations that create unnecessary chances for injury.

Athletes & Weightlifting Technique

In the world of competitive weightlifting, there is only one goal: to snatch and clean & jerk as much weight as possible. To this end, lifters often adopt certain technical practices to maximize this ability that may be inappropriate for athletes training for other sports.

When determining how to teach the lifts to athletes, what exactly is trying to be accomplished needs to be kept in mind.

The primary focus is on developing explosive leg and hip extension and the ability to safely and effectively absorb force. Any technical style that places extreme emphasis on either hip extension or leg extension and compromises the other limits the athlete's development of the traits that will improve sporting performance.

The technical style presented in this book is not always identical to what even my own competitive weightlifters are taught—it is intended specifically to be maximally productive for athletes outside the weightlifting community. This should be kept in mind if ever comparing the performance of the lifts by yourself or your athletes to that of competitive weightlifters.

Related & Substitute Exercises

The following are a few exercises that can complement the Olympic lifts in training, or in some cases replace them if the classic lifts and their more direct variants are not accessible for whatever reasons.

Clean Pull & Snatch Pull

Aside from the competition lifts themselves and squats, snatch and clean pulls are the most common training exercises in weightlifting. For the athlete, they can provide some of the training effect of the Olympic lifts, but also have unique benefits.

A pull is simply the phase of the clean or snatch in which the athlete pulls the bar from the floor and finishes with complete knee and hip extension—that is, it's a snatch or clean without any attempt to pull down under the bar. These can be loaded more heavily that snatches or cleans, and can also be done in a number of different ways to have varying effects.

The primary benefits of pulls are strengthening the legs and hips, developing explosiveness in the legs and hips, developing upper back strength and mass, and if no straps are used, strengthening the grip. High-pulls will also help develop strength and mass in the arms and shoulders along with the upper back.

Pulls can also be done from different hang positions or be started on blocks. For example, clean pulls from blocks at knee height will allow an athlete to train hip and knee explosiveness with heavier weights even if he or she is not flexible enough to lift properly from the floor or even to perform a clean of any kind with reasonable loading.

The athlete will begin in the clean or snatch starting position. After tightening the position, he or she will push with the legs to begin moving the bar, keeping the back arched and continuing to push the bar back toward the body. As the bar reaches mid to upper-thigh, the athlete will explode at the hips while continuing to forcefully push against the floor with the legs. This push with the legs will continue until the bar stops moving upward. At the top of the knee and hip extension, the athlete can shrug to give the bar

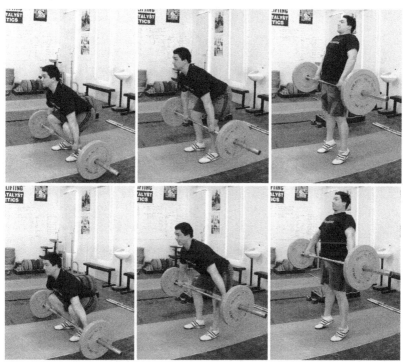

Top: clean pull; bottom: snatch pull

somewhere to go. Snatch pulls will be more difficult for the legs because of the lower starting position, but will allow more speed at the top because of the bar's position in the hips.

Athletes can use straps when performing pulls to ensure that grip is not a limiter to the weight and speed of the exercise.

Clean High-Pull & Snatch High-Pull

The high-pull differs from the pull only in the final moment after the knees and hips have finished extending. Rather than only shrugging at the top, the athlete will actively pull with the arms, lifting the elbows up and to the sides as they would when pulling down under a clean, but here the legs will continue pushing against the ground and therefore the arms will pull the bar up. Obviously the athlete will not be able to use as much weight for high-pulls as for standard pulls.

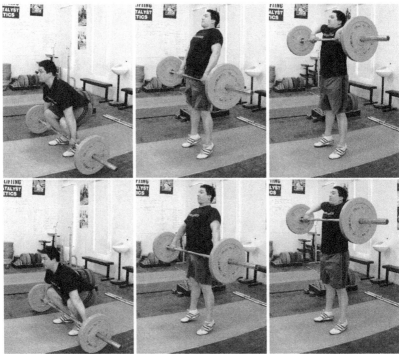

Top: clean high-pull; bottom: snatch high-pull

Jerks Behind the Neck

All jerk-related exercises can be performed with the bar starting behind the neck. This provides a strong, stable and comfortable rack position, and many athletes will be able to lift more from this starting position than they can from the front. Jerks from behind the neck may also be more accessible to athletes with limited wrist flexibility, although they do require good shoulder mobility. When performing multiple reps, athletes need to be careful lowering the bar to bring it down onto the traps rather than the neck.

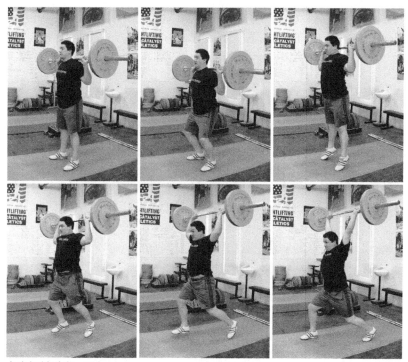

Jerk behind the neck

Jump Squat

Easily the simplest form of a loaded explosive exercise is the jump squat, of which there are many variations. First, the jump squat can be done with different squat depths. Most common is a partial squat that will be more similar to jump mechanics; less common but also useful is a full depth squat with an attempt to accelerate right away from the bottom position. The exercise can be done with a static start in the bottom position, or with a countermovement starting in a standing position. Loading for the jump squat will not be extremely heavy—the goal is explosiveness, not strength.

The jump squat can be loaded in a number of ways. The simplest is a barbell in the back squat position. This should be reserved for lighter weights or more experienced athletes who are good at stabilizing the trunk. The bar needs to be actively pulled down into the traps with the arms to prevent it from shifting and bouncing.

The athlete can also hold a pair of dumbbells on the shoulders or at arms' length, or use a trap bar. If using a trap bar, the athlete should not use straps in case a quick bailout is necessary.

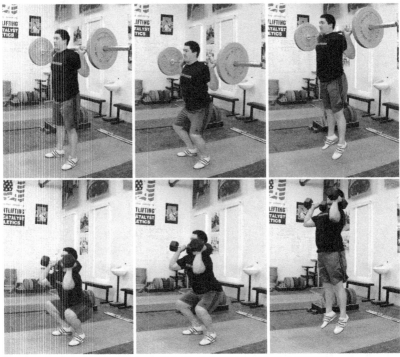

Top: quarter jump squat with barbell; bottom: jump squat with dumbbells

GREG EVERETT

The Basics of Program Design

A complete discussion of program design for athletic strength & conditioning is well beyond the scope of this book. Athletes and coaches need to design programming to be appropriate for both their sports and the individual in question. The goal here is to get the reader started with incorporating the Olympic lifts into their training programs effectively.

Sets & Reps

Most often, the Olympic lifts should be done with 3 or fewer reps. After 3 reps, fatigue, both physical and mental, will typically begin to negatively affect lift technique and speed. Higher volume can be achieved through more sets to better preserve lift quality. How many sets are used will depend on the goal for the exercise, the total training volume appropriate for the athlete at that time, and the loading. Generally speaking, 5-10 sets at the working weight will be appropriate.

Intensity

Intensity refers to the percentage of the athlete's 1 rep max in the exercise. Most athletes will not have established 1RMs for the Olympic lifts, so prescribing percentages will not always be possible. However, percentages can still be used as guides for effort.

Maximal power production occurs in the 70-80% of 1RM range where there is the ideal balance between speed and loading. Heavier loading slows the movement and reduces power; lighter loading doesn't provide enough resistance for significant power. This doesn't mean that loading outside this range does not have utility; it can be used for other goals such as technical or speed training or pushing the strength end of the spectrum more.

Frequency

How often an athlete performs the Olympic lifts can vary considerably depending on the sport, the time in the season, the training experience of the athlete, and the particular strengths and weaknesses of the athlete. Two days per week can be considered a default frequency for most athletes. One of these days can be loaded more heavily, and the other can be lighter with a focus on speed; or one day can be a pull-oriented lift like the power clean and the other day can be a push-oriented lift like the power jerk.

Strength Work

The strength basics like the back squat, front squat, deadlift, press, bench press, pull-up and bent row generally should not be replaced by Olympic lifts, although the Olympic lifts may occupy some of the volume previously occupied by accessory work or surplus strength exercise volume.

Progression

How weights and volume progress through a training cycle will depend on a number of factors, such as the length of the cycle, the point in the competitive season, and the athlete's abilities. A good rule of thumb is to increase weights for no more than 3 weeks at a time before inserting a recovery week of slightly reduced loading and significantly reduced volume.

Depending on how the cycle is constructed, the sets and reps may remain the same or nearly so while the weights are increased; more commonly, volume will be reduced as weights increase primarily through a reduction in the number of reps per set. For longer cycles, the volume may stay approximately the same in a given 3-4 week block of training, then reduce with each subsequent block; for example, in a 12-week cycle, the athlete may perform 6 reps in the squat in the first 4 weeks, 4 reps in the second 4-weeks, and 2-3 reps in the final 4 weeks (this is ignoring a recovery week in those 4-week blocks in which reps will likely be lower), with the weights increasing for the first 3 weeks of each block, then reducing slightly during the fourth week.

Another simple and common way to modulate intensity and volume is to increase weights for 2 weeks, insert a recovery week, then push the weights to max efforts or near max efforts on the fourth week. This progression would also work in the above described 12-week cycle, and in this case, the final week might be used to test 1 rep maxes.

Sample Programs

Following are two examples of program design as it pertains to the Olympic lifts in an overall program. These examples include only the Olympic lifts and some basic strength work; these are not intended to be complete training programs, although each would function effectively as an abbreviated program for an athlete with limited training time or recovery capacity.

The final sample program is an example of a complete 12-week training cycle not including conditioning and sport-specific training. This is a simple demonstration of one way of prescribing weights, sets and reps. This basic progression has been used successfully at Catalyst Athletics in many iterations. For most non-strength athletes, strength programming does not need to be exceedingly complicated, and in such cases, simplicity makes the coach's job easier and often is more effective than more complicated programming.

3-DAY TEMPLATE

Day	Exercise Type	Exercises	Sets	Reps
1	Heavy Olympic Lift	Power Clean Clean	5-10	1-3
	Squat	Back squat Front Squat	3-6	3-6
2	Push Olympic Lift	Power Jerk Split Jerk	5-10	1-3
	Upper Body Push	Bench Press Press Push Press	3-6	5-8
	Upper Body Pull	Bent Row Weighted Pull-up	3-6	5-8
3	Light Olympic Lift	Hang Power Snatch Power Snatch Hang Power Clean Power Clean	5-10	2-3
	Heavy Pull*	Snatch Pull Clean Pull Deadlift	3-6	2-5

* From floor, blocks or hang

2-DAY TEMPLATE

Day	Exercise Type	Exercises	Sets	Reps
1	Light or Push Olympic Lift	Hang Power Snatch Power Snatch Hang Power Clean Power Clean Power Jerk Split Jerk	5-10	2-3
	Squat	Back squat Front Squat	3-6	3-6
2	Heavy Olympic Lift	Power Clean Clean	5-10	1-3
	Upper Body Push	Bench Press Press Push Press	3-6	5-8
	Upper Body Pull	Bent Row Weighted Pull-up	3-6	5-8

Sample Complete Program

The following program is an example of exercise selection and set, rep and intensity prescription over the course of a 12-week training cycle. This basic template can be shortened, extended and otherwise modified fairly easily. Different exercises can be used in place of what is prescribed here to address the needs of the individual athlete, or Olympic lift variants can be changed to be appropriate for the athlete's present ability and mobility (e.g. changing power cleans to hang power cleans, or replacing snatches with cleans).

Conditioning and sport-specific skill work would generally be placed in greatest volume in the days between these strength training days, and depending on the sport, athlete and activity, may be done before or after the strength training sessions as well.

Abdominal work is done every training day. It's recommended to alternate among different types of ab work each session to ensure complete development and to keep athletes more engaged through variety. Ab work can be broken up into basic categories like trunk flexion, trunk lateral flexion, trunk rotation and static holds. Usually 3-5 sets of 10-30 reps is sufficient unless an athlete is particularly weak in this respect. In such cases, planks may be a good idea for every session before any other ab work.

Upper body accessory work can also be varied each week and usually can be left to the athlete to choose; however, it's a good idea to keep an eye on the athletes to make sure they don't simply always do the exercises they like most because those will usually be the ones they need the least. These exercises should be chosen to address hypertrophy or small muscle or movement strength. For example, an athlete who has poor scapular stability should choose upper body pull exercises that involve scapular retraction.

The program shows testing of 1 rep max for certain exercises. This should be done judiciously. If an athlete is not technically sound enough to lift a maximal effort, he or she can instead perform 3-5 sets of heavy singles.

In cases in which no weights are assigned, the numbers are sets x reps (e.g. 3 x 8 is 3 sets of 8 reps). In cases in which weights are assigned, the numbers are weight (or percentage) x reps x sets (e.g. 65% x 8 x 3 is 3 sets of 8 reps at 65%).

Note that while percentages are prescribed in most cases, these may need to be adjusted for certain athletes based on how adapted they are this type of training, how accurate the 1RMs used for calculation are, and how technically sound their lifts are. In some cases, the athlete will not have an established 1RM in a given exercise. In these instances, the percentages can be used as a guide for the desired level of effort and will show the basic progression of intensity over the course of the cycle. If the athlete is technically proficient enough, he or she can test a 1RM at the end of the cycle for use in the next one.

SAMPLE 12-WEEK PROGRAM

	Week 1	Week 2	Week 3	Week 4	Week 5	Week 6
Day 1						
Power Clean	70% x 3 x 8	75% x 3 x 6	80% x 2 x 8	85% x 2 x 6	90% x 1 x 5	Test 1RM
Back Squat	65% x 8 x 3	75% x 5 x 4	80% x 4 x 4	85% 3 x 3	90% x 1 x 3	Test 1RM
SLDL	3 x 8	3 x 8	3 x 6	3 x 6	3 x 5	3 x 5
Upper Body Pull Accessory	3-5 x 8-12	3-5 x 8-12	3-5 x 8-12	3-5 x 8-12	3-5 x 8-12	3-5 x 8-12
Abs	3-5 x 10-30	3-5 x 10-30	3-5 x 10-30	3-5 x 10-30	3-5 x 10-30	3-5 x 10-30
Day 2						
Power Jerk Behind Neck	70% x 3 x 8	75% x 3 x 6	80% x 2 x 8	85% x 2 x 6	90% x 1 x 5	Test 1RM
Bench Press	65% x 8 x 3	75% x 5 x 4	80% x 4 x 4	85% 3 x 3	90% x 1 x 3	Test 1RM
Bent Row	4 x 8	4 x 8	4 x 6	4 x 6	3 x 5	3 x 5
Upper Body Push & Pull Accessory - Vertical	3-5 x 8-12	3-5 x 8-12	3-5 x 8-12	3-5 x 8-12	3-5 x 8-12	3-5 x 8-12
Abs	3-5 x 10-30	3-5 x 10-30	3-5 x 10-30	3-5 x 10-30	3-5 x 10-30	3-5 x 10-30
Day 3						
Hang Power Snatch	70% x 3 x 8	75% x 3 x 6	80% x 2 x 8	85% x 2 x 6	90% x 1 x 5	Test 1RM
Clean Pull	5 x 5	5 x 5	5 x 4	5 x 4	5 x 3	5 x 3
Good Morning	3 x 8	3 x 8	3 x 6	3 x 6	3 x 5	3 x 5
Lunge	3 x 10	3 x 10	3 x 10	3 x 8	3 x 8	3 x 8
Upper Body Push Accessory	3-5 x 8-12	3-5 x 8-12	3-5 x 8-12	3-5 x 8-12	3-5 x 8-12	3-5 x 8-12
Abs	3-5 x 10-30	3-5 x 10-30	3-5 x 10-30	3-5 x 10-30	3-5 x 10-30	3-5 x 10-30

GREG EVERETT

SAMPLE 12-WEEK PROGRAM

	Week 7	Week 8	Week 9	Week 10	Week 11	Week 12
Day 1						
Power Clean	70% x 3 x 8	75% x 3 x 6	80% x 2 x 8	85% x 2 x 6	90% x 1 x 5	Test 1RM
Front Squat	65% x 6 x 4	75% x 5 x 4	80% x 4 x 4	85% 3 x 3	90% x 1 x 3	Test 1RM
SLDL	3 x 5	3 x 5	3 x 5	3 x 5	2 x 5	2 x 5
Upper Body Push Accessory	3-5 x 8-12	3-5 x 8-12	3-5 x 8-12	3-5 x 8-12	3-5 x 8-12	3-5 x 8-12
Abs	3-5 x 10-30	3-5 x 10-30	3-5 x 10-30	3-5 x 10-30	3-5 x 10-30	3-5 x 10-30
Day 2						
Split Jerk	70% x 3 x 8	75% x 3 x 6	80% x 2 x 8	85% x 2 x 6	90% x 1 x 5	Test 1RM
Push Press	65% x 8 x 3	75% x 5 x 4	80% x 4 x 4	85% 3 x 3	90% x 1 x 3	Test 1RM
Weighted Pull-up	4 x 10	4 x 8	5 x 6	4 x 6	3 x 5	3 x 3
Upper Body Push & Pull Accessory - Horizontal	3-5 x 8-12	3-5 x 8-12	3-5 x 8-12	3-5 x 8-12	3-5 x 8-12	3-5 x 8-12
Abs	3-5 x 10-30	3-5 x 10-30	3-5 x 10-30	3-5 x 10-30	3-5 x 10-30	3-5 x 10-30
Day 3						
Snatch	70% x 3 x 8	75% x 3 x 6	80% x 2 x 8	85% x 2 x 6	90% x 1 x 5	Test 1RM
Clean High-Pull	5 x 5	5 x 5	5 x 4	5 x 4	5 x 3	5 x 3
Good Morning	3 x 5	3 x 5	3 x 5	3 x 5	3 x 5	3 x 5
Lunge	3 x 10	3 x 10	3 x 10	3 x 8	3 x 8	3 x 8
Upper Body Pull Accessory	3-5 x 8-12	3-5 x 8-12	3-5 x 8-12	3-5 x 8-12	3-5 x 8-12	3-5 x 8-12
Abs	3-5 x 10-30	3-5 x 10-30	3-5 x 10-30	3-5 x 10-30	3-5 x 10-30	3-5 x 10-30

FLEXIBILITY

Inflexibility in the ankles, hips, thoracic spine, shoulders and wrists will limit an athlete's ability to perform the Olympic lifts and unnecessarily create opportunity for injury. However, with limited training time and so many other athletic traits in need of development, along with the general unpleasantness of stretching, flexibility is often neglected by athletes and coaches.

The goal for the coach and athlete is to address flexibility as needed with as little time commitment as possible. Limiting the time commitment means both keeping the amount of time dedicated to flexibility work in a given training session to as little as needed to be effective, but also ensuring that improvements are made as quickly as possible to allow the reduction of flexibility work as an athlete's career progresses. It takes far less time and effort to maintain a given level of flexibility than to achieve it.

Flexibility is ideally developed very early in the process of athletic development along with other general physical traits that create the foundation for athletic specialization, but the majority of athletes will arrive in a training program with less than optimal flexibility. This then needs to be addressed along with the other training elements to ensure safe training and maximal development.

Optimal Flexibility

Each athlete will require a certain degree of mobility in each joint to optimize performance in his or her sport. The demands on flexibility can vary greatly among sports, and excessive flexibility is only somewhat less problematic than inadequate flexibility. Coaches will need to determine what is appropriate for their athletes based on the requirements of the sport.

Specifically for the performance of the Olympic lifts, athletes need to be able to safely and comfortably achieve the proper positions in the following:

- Front Squat (below parallel minimum)
- Overhead Squat (below parallel minimum)
- Jerk Rack Position
- Jerk Overhead Position (power and split)
- Snatch and Clean Start Position

Front Squat

In order to safely perform the clean, an athlete must be able to sit into a structurally sound front squat position to at least immediately below parallel in depth. Ideally an athlete can achieve a full-depth front squat (i.e. fully closed knee joint), but for most non-weightlifter athletes, this is beyond reasonable expectation. For athletes who will only be performing power cleans, the necessary

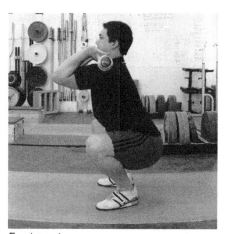

Front squat

front squat position will be only a partial squat (above parallel). Irrespective of the necessary depth, the rack position of the barbell must be equally sound. This means the bar is supported directly by the trunk on the shoulders, not by the hands and arms. With the feet flat on the floor and the lifter balanced, the lower back must be extended and the trunk upright.

Overhead Squat

To perform the snatch, an athlete must be capable of achieving a structurally sound overhead squat to at least immediately below parallel depth. Inadequate flexibility in this position opens the athlete up to possible shoulder, elbow and wrist injury in particular. For athletes who will be performing only power snatches, the necessary overhead squat position will be only a partial squat

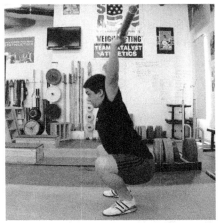
Overhead squat

(above parallel). With the feet flat and the lifter balanced, the lower back must be extended, the trunk upright, the shoulder blades retracted, the elbows fully extended, and the barbell over the base of the neck.

Jerk Rack Position

For an athlete to perform an effective jerk or push press, a solid position of the bar on the shoulders with the arms in a good position to press against the bar is necessary. Such a position will also reduce the stress to the wrists and elbows. The shoulders must be pushed forward and slightly up with the bar resting solidly on top; the bar

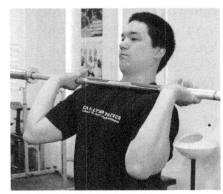
Jerk rack position

should be as deep in the palms as possible and the elbows spread out to the sides and slightly in front of the bar.

Jerk Overhead Position

The athlete must be able to achieve a sound position in either a split or power receiving position (depending on which variation is used) with a jerk grip to ensure safety for the shoulders, elbows, wrists and lower back in particular. The barbell should be over the base of the neck with the shoulder blades retracted and the elbows fully extended.

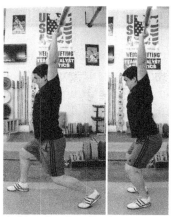

Jerk overhead position

Snatch & Clean Starting Position

If the athlete will be pulling snatches or cleans from the floor, the flexibility to set a proper back arch at the appropriate knee and hip angles is necessary for safe and effective lifting. With the feet flat and the bar over the balls of the feet, the athlete should be able to arch the back with the shoulders directly over the bar or slightly in front of it.

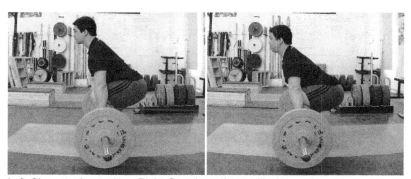

Left: Clean starting position; Right: Snatch starting position

Mobility vs. Flexibility

Once an athlete has achieved the necessary degree of flexibility through static stretching, it will generally be possible to maintain it with little or no further static stretching. Performing movements through the full range of motion, along with dynamic mobility work during warm-ups, will maintain the necessary range of motion very well. A notable exception to this is periods of heavy, high-volume training, particularly with a considerable hypertrophy component. The attendant muscular growth and soreness and stiffness can reduce flexibility again over time if the athlete fails to actively maintain it. It's recommended that during such periods of training, the athlete return to performing enough static stretching at the end of training sessions to maintain flexibility.

Timing of Stretching

With the exception of selected stretches that are necessarily done prior to training to allow an athlete to achieve positions to lift safely, static stretching should be reserved for the post-training window to prevent any possible temporary nerve disruption that could reduce power output or proprioception during training. Once stretches are selected for an athlete, an ideal order of performance should be determined that allows a natural flow from stretch to stretch to maximize economy. This will minimize time investment to allow it to fit in a tight training schedule and make it more likely that the athlete will continue with the flexibility program.

Another method of minimizing the time demands of stretching is to perform certain stretches between sets of lifting exercises. This should be done discriminately to avoid stretching muscles or in ways that will disrupt the following set. Unless the stretching is needed to improve the athlete's position in the exercise in question (and in such cases, it should be done prior to that exercise rather than during), it's generally wise to stretch unrelated body parts. For example, performing shoulder girdle stretches between sets of squats will save time, but will not create any potential problems by performing static stretches of muscles that will immediately need to generate force.

Stretches

The following stretches were selected because of their simplicity and effectiveness. They are by no means the only stretches available to address the muscle groups in question, but they will be sufficient for the majority of athletes. If additional stretches are determined necessary, athletes and coaches are encouraged to experiment to find what works best.

Static stretches can be held for 20-60 seconds as needed. PNF stretching can be performed where possible to speed results: After holding an initial stretch for 20-30 seconds, the athlete will isometrically activate the muscle being stretched at about a 20% effort against the resistance for 5-6 seconds, then relax and increase the stretch gently for 5-6 seconds. This contract-relax alternation should be repeated 5-6 times, then followed with a final static stretch for 20-30 seconds.

The stretches are grouped according to the positions they can be used to help improve. Note that there is of course some crossover among some of them. Consider also that certain positions involve more than one group. For example, the overhead squat requires squat-related flexibility along with overhead-related flexibility.

Squat & Starting Position

The following stretches will help increase flexibility of the ankles and hips primarily, which will allow athletes to squat deeper with the proper posture, as well as achieve sound starting positions for the snatch and clean with properly extended backs.

Ankle Stretch

Sitting in a squat position, lean the forearms on one knee to close the ankle. Keep the foot flat on the floor. If the ankles are very inflexible, this position might not be accessible; an alternative is to perform the stretch from a lunge position instead.

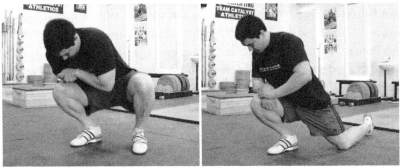

Left: squatting ankle stretch; Right: lunging ankle stretch

Russian Baby Maker

With the feet somewhat wider than the normal squat stance and the feet turned out only slightly, place the hands on top of the feet, bend the arms and push the elbows into the insides of the thighs as deep toward the hips as possible. Push the elbows out as you sit down on the arms, spreading the thighs where they attach to the hip. Remember that this stretch is not spreading the knees; it's spreading the hips.

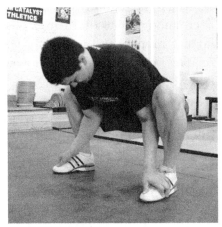

Russian baby maker

Spiderman Lunge

Take a long lunge step and lean down to push the trunk as far down below the lead leg as possible. Take a long lunge step and lean down to push the trunk as far down below the lead leg as possible. Push the hips down along with the chest. Bending the front knee less will increase the intensity of the stretch.

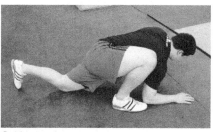
Spiderman lunge

Lying Hamstring

The ideal way to stretch the hamstrings is in a supine lying position that allows the athlete to maintain the natural arch of the lower back and ensure the movement is actually occurring at the hip rather than the lumbar spine. Lying on the back, ideally with a thin towel roll or similar under the lower back to support the arch, the athlete will loop a stretching strap around the foot and pull the leg back, keeping the other leg straight and flat on the floor to prevent the hips from rolling back.

The athlete should contract the quad during the stretch both to keep the knee straight and to encourage the hamstrings to relax. This stretch can be changed to target the hamstrings differently as needed by pulling the leg slightly inward or outward rather than straight back. It can also be done with a bent knee. This is a perfect stretch to use the PNF contract-relax protocol with.

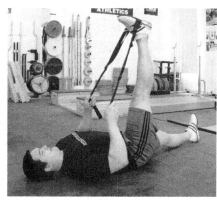
Lying hamstring stretch

Jerk & Clean Rack Position

The following stretches can be used to address flexibility limitations for the clean and jerk rack positions. They will help athletes place the barbell properly on the shoulders with the hands open and elbows up for the clean, and with the bar in the palm and elbows down and out for the jerk. Note that the first thing any athlete struggling to achieve these rack positions should do is experiment with different grip widths. Often a relative minor change in width (usually shifting wider) will offset flexibility or proportion-related limitations dramatically. Some of the stretches in the overhead position category will also help with the rack positions.

Wrist Flexor Stretches

Before doing any wrist stretches, it's a good idea to decompress the joint by shaking the hands and pulling the hand straight out away from the forearm for some traction.

The most basic wrist and finger flexor stretch can be done simply using one hand to push against the other in front of the body. The hand can also be pressed against a wall, the floor or a power rack to allow the stretch to be done with a straight elbow. Changing the orientation of the hand (e.g. fingers up, down or to one side) will change the stretch somewhat.

To stretch the wrist and include the thumb, the fingers can be pressed against the safety pin of a power rack with the thumb against the upright.

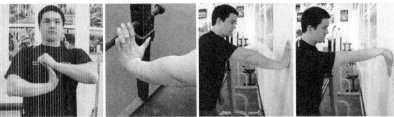

Left to right: Basic finger and wrist flexor stretch; wrist stretch with thumb; wrist stretch on wall with fingers up and down.

Rack Elevators

Both the clean and jerk rack positions can be stretched with rack elevators. Place a loaded barbell in a squat rack, squat partially with the feet under the bar and position the hands in the appropriate way for the rack position being stretched, then stand, using the legs to push the shoulders up into the bar while maintaining the proper hand and arm positions. For the clean rack, a partner can also push the elbows up for the athlete when in this position.

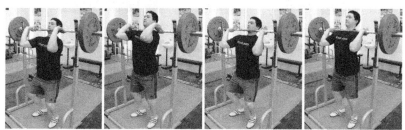

Left: Clean rack elevator start and finish; Right: Jerk rack elevator start and finish.

Scapular Protraction

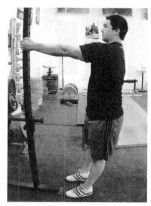

Necessary to achieving either rack position is the ability to protract the scapulae considerably. A simple stretch is to stand in front of a power rack, grip the upright with one arm, and lean the body back away from the rack, keeping the chest squared off straight ahead. The athlete needs to maintain extension of the upper back rather than allowing it to round forward as will be natural.

Scapular protraction

Burgener Rack Stretch

This stretch comes from Mike Burgener. With a clean grip on the bar, the athlete will place the bar behind the neck as he or she would for a back squat, then lift the elbows forward and up as much as possible. This can be done with both a closed and open grip. The grip can be moved wider to shift more of the stretch to the scapular area, which will help the jerk rack position more. The shoulders should be elevated slightly and pushed forward as much as possible in both variations of the stretch.

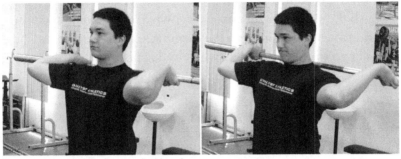

Burgener bar stretch close and wide grip

Snatch & Jerk Overhead Position

The following set of stretches will address flexibility for the overhead positions of the snatch and jerk. It should be kept in mind that in the snatch, poor hip and especially ankle flexibility, or thoracic spine immobility, can appear to be limited shoulder mobility because the athlete is attempting to bring the arms into position while on an improper base and consequently demanding excessive range of motion from the shoulders.

Thoracic Spine Foam Rolling

Critical to increasing overhead range of motion is ensuring proper mobility of the thoracic spine. Part of every athlete's warm-up should be foam rolling of the upper back, particularly those with limited overhead range of motion. With the foam roller perpendicular to the spine, the athlete will lie on his or her back and roll up and down the thoracic spine, trying to relax the back around the curve of the roller. Initially the athlete can fold the arms across the chest loosely, but rolling can also be done with the arms overhead. The athlete can also simply lie on the roller and allow the upper back to settle down around it, moving along the thoracic spine every 10-30 seconds.

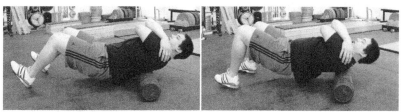

Thoracic spine foam rolling

Doorjamb Shoulder Girdle Stretch

This a simple and very effective stretch for the shoulder girdle. The athlete will place the forearm vertically against a doorjamb or the upright of a power rack. The elbow should be bent and higher than the shoulder; the height can be adjusted to change the direction of the stretch somewhat. The athlete will lean and push the chest forward.

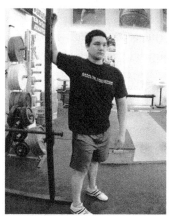

Door jamb shoulder girdle stretch

Leaning Bar Hang

This is a modification to the basic hang from a bar to improve the stretch. The athlete will grip a pull-up bar with the hands outside shoulder width (usually approximately clean-width grip) and hang from the bar with the toes touching the floor several inches behind the bar. A plyo box or similar can be used for the toes as

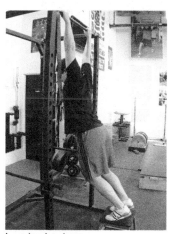

Leaning bar hang

needed to account for height. This will allow the athlete to hang most of his or her bodyweight, but the contact with the toes will allow somewhat more relaxation, usually allow easier breathing, and by placing the toes behind the bar, will help open the shoulders more than with a direct vertical hang.

Doorjamb Underarm Stretch

This stretch will address the muscles that attach under the upper arm and help the shoulder open more. With the elbow bent, the athlete will place the underside of the upper arm near the elbow against a doorjamb or the upright of a power rack with the body squared off facing the door or rack. He or she will lean forward to bring the elbow back over the shoulder, not allowing it to move out to the side significantly. The free hand can be

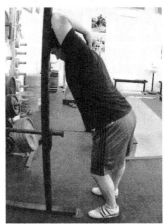

Doorjamb underarm stretch

used to push the forearm somewhat to help keep the arm being stretched squared off properly.

CATALYST ATHLETICS

Find more information on Oympic weightlifting from
Catalyst Athletics, including articles, training and
instructional videos, books, DVDs and posters.

www.catalystathletics.com

WANT MORE?

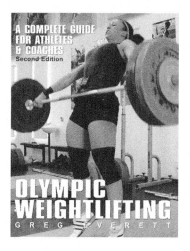

Olympic Weightlifting: A Complete Guide for Athletes & Coaches is a comprehensive guide to learning and instructing the Olympic and related lifts. Includes sections on learning progressions, lift analyses, error correction, competition, programming, sample training programs, flexibility, warm-up protocols, and nutrition.

Paperback; 423 pages; 8.5" x 11"

Available at **catalystathletics.com** and other book retailers.

"Simply the best book available on Olympic weightlifting." —*Don Weideman, Vice President, Pacific Weightlifting Association*

"Without a doubt the best book on the market today about Olympic-style weightlifting." —*Mike Burgener, USA Weightlifting senior international coach*

"Outstanding, Accurate, and Concise! A must read for athletes and coaches involved in the movements." —*Daniel Camargo, USA Weightlifting International Coach; President, Florida Weightlifting Federation*

"Everett's Olympic Weightlifting text is one of the best instructional books for the sport to be published in years. This is a must have for every weightlifting/ strength and conditioning coach's library shelf." —*Bob Takano, Member USA Weightlifting Hall of Fame*

"Everett's book is one of the most accessible and comprehensive weightlifting sources available for the coach and athlete today. I highly recommend this book for every serious strength coach or weightlifting practitioner." —*John Thrush, Head Coach Calpians Weightlifting*

"This is the book I would recommend to anyone wanting to begin the sport of Weightlifting. Greg took material that has been discussed for decades by many many great coaches and authors and managed to present it with a clarity that has rarely, if ever, been achieved. Greg has a way of taking material that has been argued and discussed to death, and presenting it in such a clear way that it makes you wonder why anything else ever had to be written or said." —*Glenn Pendlay, Head Coach, California Strength Weightlifting Team*

Made in the USA
Coppell, TX
26 August 2021

61078425R00069